INTERCULTURAL PERSPECTIVES ON FAMILY COUNSELING

Intercultural Perspectives on Family Counseling expands cultural awareness in the practice of family counseling by offering cultural-specific perspectives for addressing common issues that emerge in dyadic, marital, and family relationships around the globe.

The topics illuminated in the book serve to sharpen cultural mindfulness and expand the reader's knowledge and understanding of intercultural family counseling issues. Each chapter examines a couple or family-related clinical issue, offering clinical intervention strategies within the context of a specific cultural population. By representing various national and cultural identities, this book showcases a transcultural understanding of family.

Students and practicing marriage and family counselors and therapists will benefit greatly from this clinical resource that exposes them to the similarities and differences in addressing client issues across cultures.

Brian S. Canfield is Professor of Clinical Mental Health Counseling at Florida Atlantic University, USA.

FAMILY SYSTEMS COUNSELING: INNOVATIONS THEN AND NOW

Series Editor: Paul R. Peluso, PhD, Florida Atlantic University

This series is aimed at both current practitioners and students who wish to learn about the historical power and boldness of the family systems approach, but who also need to see it applied to current problem situations. The books in this series will reflect on the pioneering elements of family systems approaches and how they might have been used previously with a particular issue or population.

Intercultural Perspectives on Family Counseling
Edited by Brian S. Canfield

A Family Systems Guide to Infidelity
Helping Couples Understand, Recover From, and Avoid Future Affairs
Paul R. Peluso

For more information about this series, please visit https://www.routledge.com/Family-Systems-Counseling-Innovations-Then-and-Now/book-series/FSCTN

INTERCULTURAL PERSPECTIVES ON FAMILY COUNSELING

Edited by Brian S. Canfield

Routledge
Taylor & Francis Group
NEW YORK AND LONDON

First published 2020
by Routledge
52 Vanderbilt Avenue, New York, NY 10017

and by Routledge
2 Park Square, Milton Park, Abingdon, Oxon OX14 4RN

Routledge is an imprint of the Taylor & Francis Group, an informa business

Library of Congress Cataloging-in-Publication Data
A catalog record for this title has been requested

ISBN: 978-0-8153-7998-0 (hbk)
ISBN: 978-0-8153-7999-7 (pbk)
ISBN: 978-1-351-21438-4 (ebk)

Typeset in Bembo
by Taylor & Francis Books

CONTENTS

ILLUSTRATIONS

Tables

Boxes

SERIES EDITOR'S FOREWORD

This book, *Intercultural Perspectives on Family Counseling* by Dr. Brian Canfield is a unique text that addresses a critical need. While there are a plethora of books that address multiculturalism in counseling and psychotherapy, they tend to consider multiculturalism from a static position (one group as majority and another group as minority, and how to handle the dynamics between each), centered in North America.

Dr. Canfield has assembled a group of truly diverse authors who were challenged to look at it from a more dynamic approach where there are multiple cultural perspectives within and amongst various populations. He and his collaborators represent one of the broadest swaths of practitioners from all over the globe. They tackle specific issues and real-world problems that practitioners must deal with in a culturally sensitive and competent fashion. From Domestic Violence Counseling for couples and families in Russia to the impact of gender role negotiation with Jewish couples, this book has the potential to provide valuable information on subjects never before discussed or detailed from a clinical perspective.

In addition, understanding the intercultural issues as systems-based issues will provide a unifying framework for the reader to contextualize the clinical approaches squarely within a Family Systems Approach. Within this text, readers will be able to see how family therapy is practiced in Asia, the Middle East, Africa, Europe, and North America, negotiating the sometimes tricky aspects of differing cultural beliefs and practices, all while keeping a Systems Theory perspective towards the goal of helping couples and families live in harmony with each other. With the current state of upheaval in the world today, never has there been a book that has been needed more than this one.

Paul R. Peluso, Ph.D
August 2019

CONTRIBUTORS

Mehmet Nurullah Akkurt is a native of Saudi Arabia. He earned his Ph.D. in the United States and currently serves on the faculty of a university in Saudi Arabia.

Khalid A. Alfallatah is a Ph.D. candidate in Counselor Education and Supervision at Barry University. In addition to his teaching experience, he has held active professional leadership roles and has shared his research and clinical work at professional conferences throughout the USA and internationally. Khalid is currently the Imam at the Evergreen Islamic Institute in Seattle, WA. His research interests include Islamic Studies, psychopathology, neuro-psychotherapy, family therapy, and client resilience.

Jason P. Austin earned a Ph.D. in Family Therapy from Virginia Polytechnic Institute and State University. He is a Licensed Marriage and Family Therapist, Licensed Professional Counselor, and serves on the faculty of the University of Louisiana at Monroe as Assistant Professor in the marriage and family therapy graduate program. His clinical work utilizes an empowerment perspective to bring about positive life changes. In his work with underserved populations, he focuses on the intersection of multiple societal systems and clients' problems and advocacy.

Jamie Banker has a Ph.D. in Human Development and Marriage and Family Therapy from Virginia Polytechnic Institute and State University. She is a Licensed Marriage and Family Therapist and an AAMFT approved supervisor. Jamie is an Associate Professor at California Lutheran University and served as the Director of the Counseling Psychology-MFT Program for seven years. Her clinical and research interests are women's and family health. Her research interests include community trauma, young adult sexuality, and best practices in systemic therapy interventions.

E. Carolina Benitez was born and raised in Honduras and immigrated to the United States in 1995. She received her Ph.D. in Counselor Education and Supervision from the University of North Carolina at Charlotte. She is an Assistant Professor of Counseling and Clinical Training Coordinator at Gordon-Conwell Seminary and Clinical Director of Camino's Behavioral Health Clinic. She is also a Licensed Professional Counselor in North Carolina and a Nationally Certified Counselor with experience working in outpatient addiction programs, community counseling clinics, and private practice. Her clinical work focuses on prevention and treatment of mental health issues, and the impact of acculturation and spirituality factors on mental health.

Brian S. Canfield is Professor of Clinical Mental Health Counseling at Florida Atlantic University. He is a Licensed Psychologist, Licensed Marriage and Family Therapist, and a Licensed Professional Counselor. Brian received his B.A. in Psychology and M.A. in Counseling from Louisiana Tech University. He earned the Doctor of Education degree in Counseling and Guidance, with an emphasis in marriage and family therapy from Texas A&M University at Commerce. Dr. Canfield is a Fellow and Past President of the American Counseling Association.

Wentao Chao earned his Ph.D. in Marriage and Family Therapy from the University of Hong Kong and his M.A. degree in Marriage, Family and Child Counseling from Sonoma State University (USA). Wentao is Professor of Counselor Education at National Taipei University of Education in Taiwan. He is a Licensed Counseling Psychologist and Certified Marriage and Family Counselor. He has held numerous national leadership roles and has been a practicing counselor, specializing in work with couples and families for over 20 years. In addition to his clinical and university work, Dr. Chao is active as a trainer and workshop presenter internationally.

Ruoxi Chen received her Ph.D. from Virginia Polytechnic Institute and State University. She is Assistant Professor of Marriage and Family Therapy at the University of Louisiana at Monroe. She teaches practice and research courses in marriage and family therapy to master's and doctoral students. Her main research interests include relationship education, mate selection, family dynamics, and cross-cultural comparisons.

Ashley Cooper is a Licensed Mental Health Counselor in the State of Florida. She earned her Master of Science in Applied Psychology from Lynn University and is a Ph.D. candidate in Counselor Education and Supervision at Florida Atlantic University. Ashley has worked in various clinical settings including private practice with couples, children, and individuals. Her research interests include intimate partner violence and the mental health impact of gender inequality.

Neda Deylami is a native of Iran. She earned her Ph.D. degree from the University of Putra Malaysia. Dr. Deylami currently resides in Malaysia and serves as a family counselor at the Association of Family Studies in Kuala Lumpur.

Benjamin J. Evans is a Ph.D. student in Marriage and Family Therapy at the University of Louisiana at Monroe.

Susan J. Foster holds a doctoral degree and is Associate Professor at the Chicago School of Professional Psychology. She practices counseling and supervision in the state of Louisiana. Her professional experience is in community mental health, partial hospitalization units, private practice, and the K-12 school setting. Her areas of specialization include working with individuals and families who are struggling with grief, trauma, eco-anxiety, marginalization, and trafficking. She is also a subject matter expert in supervision, as well as ethics, law, and advocacy for underserved populations.

Daniel Gutierrez received his Ph.D. at the University of Central Florida. He is an Assistant Professor in the Counselor Education program at William & Mary College in Williamsburg, Virginia. He is a Licensed Professional Counselor in several states with experience working with individuals, families, and couples in various clinical settings. His research focuses on serving the underserved, especially Latinx individuals.

Jarodd W. Hundley is a Ph.D. student in Marriage and Family Therapy at the University of Louisiana at Monroe. He has worked with domestic violence, substance abuse, and family issues. His research and clinical interests include services to low socioeconomic client populations, reintegration of soldiers and their families after deployment, post-traumatic stress disorders, and cultural competence and diversity.

Berke Kirikkanat earned her B.A. in psychology from Boğaziçi University and received her Ph.D. in guidance and counseling from Marmara University. She is an Assistant Professor in the Department of Guidance and Counseling at Yeditepe University. She has conducted research on diverse topics, including attachment styles, future time orientations in romantic relationships, loneliness, irrational beliefs, marriage burn-out, subjective well-being, interpersonal cognitive distortions, academic achievement, psychological capital, academic coping strategies, academic confidence, career planning, emotional intelligence, and cognitive flexibility.

Fotini Kranou Kyriakides earned her Ph.D. in Psychology from the University of Cyprus. She works as a Collaborative Academic Staff at Frederick University Cyprus in the Psychology and Social Work Department. In her professional career she has worked as Head of the Student Development Center of Cyprus University of Technology and as Head of the Counseling Office of University of Cyprus, at the Cyprus Family Welfare Services, and as a clinician at various settings like correctional facilities and war veteran support agencies in the USA, at rehabilitation hospitals, and in the private sector in Cyprus.

Irene Leblanc holds an M.A. in Marriage and Family Therapy from the University of Louisiana at Monroe and a Ph.D. in Counselor Education and

Supervision from Florida Atlantic University. Her doctoral dissertation examined treatment and recovery issues for females with an identified substance use disorder. Irene is a Licensed Mental Health Counselor in the State of Florida and a Licensed Marriage and Family Therapist in the State of Louisiana. She works in the field of substance abuse treatment in south Florida.

Stephen E. May is a student in the Ph.D. program in Marriage and Family Therapy at the University of Louisiana at Monroe. He has a B.A. and an M.S. in Psychology, as well as a Post-graduate Certificate in Gerontology. In his clinical work, he works with diverse populations, with a particular interest in helping older clients struggling with symptoms of dementia and the impact upon families.

Miriam Moreno-Duany is a Licensed Mental Health Counselor in the State of Florida. Miriam is completing her Ph.D. degree in Counselor Education and Supervision at Florida Atlantic University. She earned her Master of Science in Mental Health Counseling from Johns Hopkins University and a Bachelor of Arts from the University of Maryland, Baltimore County. A native of Cuba, her clinical expertise includes multicultural family issues. Her research interests include chronic illness, Hispanic community, and marital issues. Miriam currently works with children identified on the autism spectrum.

Alena Prikhidko earned her Ph.D. in Counselor Education and Supervision from the University of Florida. She serves on the faculty of Florida International University as Assistant Professor of Counselor Education. Dr. Prikhidko has worked as a Mental Health and Marriage and Family Counselor in both Russia and the United States. She is involved in leadership and actively promotes ethical counseling practice in her home country of Russia; and has participated in establishing the Board on Ethics in Counseling Psychology in that country.

Abeer Ali Rasheed is a native of Saudi Arabia. Dr. Raheed earned her Ph.D. in the United States and currently serves on faculty at a university in Saudi Arabia.

Bethany Simmons received her Ph.D. from the University of Louisiana at Monroe in Marriage and Family Therapy and is a Licensed Marriage and Family Therapist, Licensed Professional Counselor and AAMFT Approved Supervisor. She is an Assistant Professor and former Director of Clinical Training at California Lutheran University's M.S. Counseling Psychology-MFT Program. Her current research focuses on systemic/cybernetic theory to training and supervision, as well as broader social/political/cultural around social responsibility, power, privilege, cultural diversity, and mental health practices. Her clinical work spans diverse settings working with underserved and marginalized populations in inpatient and outpatient settings.

Lori L. Soli, Ph.D. is an Associate Professor and the Director of Clinical Training for the CMHC Online campus at the Chicago School of Professional Psychology and maintains a small tele-mental health practice. She specializes in working with individuals and families with grief, trauma, wellness, aging, and in using experiential and alternative activities within the therapeutic process. She is a subject matter expert in supervision, clinical practice, and CACREP accreditation. Dr. Soli has been a counselor and educator for 25 years, has served in counselor education leadership positions in, and has presented and published nationally and internationally.

Daniel Williamson is Department Chair and Professor of Graduate Counseling at the University of Mary Hardin-Baylor. He received his Ph.D. from Baylor University, and is a Fulbright Specialist Alumnus in Mental Health. Dr. Williamson is a Licensed Professional Counselor in Texas, Licensed Professional Clinical Counselor supervisor in Kentucky, a National Certified Counselor, and a Human Services Board-certified Practitioner. Dr. Williamson is the Co-Founder of PAX Consulting and Counseling, PLLC.

Jennifer Williamson holds a Ph.D. from Baylor University. She is a Fulbright Specialist Alumna in Mental Health. She has presented nationally and internationally on counselor ethics and international issues. Dr. Williamson was the 2015 recipient of the Association for Counselor Education and Supervision's (ACES) Counseling Vision and Innovation Award and the 2017 recipient of the European Branch of the American Counseling Association's Professional Clinical Counselor of the Year Award. Dr. Williamson is the Co-Founder of PAX Consulting and Counseling, PLLC.

1

BASICS OF INTERCULTURAL FAMILY COUNSELING

Brian S. Canfield

Introduction

There are many theoretical and clinical models that may be employed by a family counselor to help a client. Most approaches are useful *with some clients, in some situations*. However, no counseling approach has been shown to be effective with *every client, in every situation*. While the field of counseling seeks to find answers to these questions, there is a paucity of clinical outcome research regarding various approaches to intercultural family counseling (Bitter, 2009). This poses a dilemma in the practice of family counseling, begging the question: *What approach works best with what type of client?* The challenge becomes more complex when considering cultural factors when working with couples and families.

An initial challenge for the family counselor is to utilize a conceptual model and therapeutic approach that maximizes the likelihood of helping the client, while minimizing any potential risk. While existing clinical outcome studies in the field provide some general guidance, given the multitude of variables and factors for consideration this remains largely an individualized process, specific to each counselor. This chapter offers some suggestions that may be helpful to a family counselor who seeks to expand their understanding of intercultural issues when working with couples and families.

Similarities and Differences

"Culture" refers to the institutions, traditions, and rituals by which collective knowledge is maintained and conveyed to subsequent generations (Canfield & Locke, 1992). A client's "cultural identity" provides a sense of commonality with others who share a similar identity based on shared values, beliefs, or attributes. At its essence, "Cultural identity" is a form of tribalism. It is by nature exclusionary, creating a sense of "us" that is separate and distinct from those who are not members of the cultural group. Cultural identity creates a commonality with some, and a sense of separateness with others (Canfield, 2018). Parsing humanity into various groups based on some quality or set of characteristics is both potentially useful and problematic. The term "Intercultural" differs from the term "multicultural" in that it emphasizes interactive parity between people of different cultural groups. This equal interaction between parties serves as the basis of a collaborative counseling relationship.

Our beliefs, values, ideas, and attitudes may evolve over the course of life due to education, life experiences, and exposure to new ideas. However, the cultural group in which we are embedded, beginning at birth, provides a "reference point" by which all other subsequent life experiences, concepts, and ideas are compared. While a person can change a belief, one can never fully escape the influences of their cultural family of origin (Canfield, 1992).

Even in so-called "open societies" that encourage or at least tolerate a wide-range of beliefs and ideas, people are still imprinted with the values of that society's predominant culture. From a post-modern perspective, the capacity for people within a particular society to "value diversity" and accept a "multitude of beliefs" – is merely a reflection of a cultural value and belief which "values diversity" and encourages the expression of "multiple perspectives." In this vein, the collective world view of one cultural group is not inherently superior to the world view of another society – it is merely different in terms of the presence and scope of specific beliefs.

By and large, a society expects its members to conform, at least within parameters, to the standards and values of that society. Communities create mechanisms to ensure that members adhere to the standards of the society. Maintaining a level of social control is a hall mark of civilization and is necessary to maintain a stable and orderly society. Individuals who deviate from the cultural values of the community often incur disfavor or punishment. A recognition of this reality has implications for the practice of family counseling within any specific cultural context.

Considering that clients who violate the rules of society may incur negative consequences, it is incumbent upon the family counselor to safeguard the welfare of clients, with regard to the societal consequences of various client actions. In terms of potential consequences, addressing the "coming out" of a gay son to his parents in south Florida is markedly different from Uganda or Saudi Arabia.

The concept of *Family* – referring to a group of individuals related by blood, marriage, or co-habitation – exists in various forms in all human societies. In various cultures, this may include monogamous and polygamous marriages with children, same sex couples, multigenerational extended families, single parent families, and remarried and blended families. *Family* is a social construct that continues to evolve and adapt to the changing trends. For example, the so-called "traditional nuclear family" has become less common in American society. The stereotypic "American family" popularized in 1950s pop culture, consisting of a married White heterosexual couple of European ancestry with two biological children in which the father was the primary economic earner and the mother was a "stay-at-home" Mom, economically "middle class," and religiously identified as "Christian," constituted less than 3% of the US population at the turn of the 21st century (McGoldrick, 1998.)

Shifting demographics and increased population mobility have changed the nature of family relationships. People from various cultural backgrounds are increasingly residing in locales outside of their communities of origin. These migratory movements – sometimes temporary, sometimes permanent – occur for a variety of reasons. Some relocations are voluntary, sought in the pursuit of greater economic opportunity or an enhanced quality of life. For others, relocation is involuntary, undertaken out of safety concerns in order to escape economic deprivation, societal instability, or conflict. Regardless of the reasons, persons from various cultural backgrounds increasingly find them themselves living in a community that is often markedly different from their culture of origin.

While the cultural "rules" may differ in terms of how life events and challenges are viewed, people from various backgrounds often experience similar life stressors. Economic challenges, work related issues, health concerns, martial or relationship conflict, parent-child issues, and the care and support of aging family members are common challenges encountered in all human societies. While humans share similar life experiences, the manifestation of those experiences differ.

As a result of the meaning we assign to our commonalities and differences, we may feel closer to some, and more distant from others. Such similarities and differences serve to form our initial impressions of others, as well as the impressions others form of us. This realization is relevant to client engagement in the counseling process.

Application of Cybernetics in Intercultural Family Counseling

While the potential benefits of *counseling* are well known to many, others may hold a differing opinion. Informed by societal biases, some people view "counseling" with caution, suspicion, even trepidation. In some groups, counseling is seen as an intrusive activity, in terms of time, effort, and cost. For example, the member of a community that places a premium on privacy or self-sufficiency may not readily understand or appreciate the well-intentioned efforts of the family counselor who asks probing or personal questions. The prospect of inviting a family counselor, an outsider, to become privy to intimate issues and secrets of the family, can be an immense barrier in seeking help.

As such, the practice of family counseling requires cultural sensitivity, in addition to professional knowledge and skill. While the utilization of an appropriate theoretical model and specific techniques are important, it is the ability to convey and demonstrate a genuine desire to "help" that will serve to transcend cultural barriers and allow the family counselor to most effectively join with the client to bring about desired changes.

A conceptual framework of cybernetics underscores the inter-relationship between the counselor and client. Applied cybernetics emphasizes the *co-constructed* nature of a therapeutic relationship, one in which each person serves as the logical complement to the role of another person within the therapeutic system (Becvar, Canfield, & Becvar, 1997). The concepts of applied cybernetics offer a model that is culturally flexible. This approach considers a number of factors, including:

- An awareness of the cultural identity of both the counselor and the client couple or family, and a sensitivity as to how cultural commonalities and differences may potentially impact the therapeutic relationship and counseling process.
- Recognition of the inter-relationship of the counseling process and the fact that the family counselor constitutes half of the therapeutic relationship. As such, family counselor "self-awareness" with regard to cultural identity and world view is recognized as a critically essential variable in counseling practice. Of particular importance is a consideration of how the family counselor's identity may be projected and perceived by the client couple or family.
- A respect for the cultural values and traditions of the client, and an on-going effort to uphold the right of the client to make choices within the context of their particular culture.
- Selecting theories, strategies, and techniques for facilitating desired changes that are best suited to the cultural context of the client.
- Gaining an understanding of how the client's personal values and beliefs are consistent with, or may differ from, the family or community cultural context in which the client is embedded.

At the core of an Applied Cybernetic approach to family counseling is the recognition that human relationships – "couples," "families," "groups," "extended families," or "therapeutic systems," – are defined and constructed by members of that relationship system. A system that includes, at least temporarily, the family counselor (Becvar et al., 1997.)

Central to this perspective is a recognition that all human roles and relationships are interactive, recursive, and self-sustaining in nature. This follows the logic that for every "role" there exists a corresponding complementary role. For example, the role of "teacher," requires the logical complement of "student." The role of "parent" requires the logical complementary role of "child." Other examples include: "seller – buyer," "lawyer – client," "thief – victim," "police officer – offender," "husband – wife," and "doctor – patient." In understanding role complementarity, it is important to recognize that one role does not necessarily *create* its logical role complement. However, a logical complement must exist in order to maintain any relational role. Remove a "bully" and no one is "bullied." This concept of *logical role complementarity* is an essential element in understanding the relational nature of the family counseling from a cybernetic perspective (Becvar et al., 1997.)

Unlike the majority of psychological theories which typically view the client as a self-contained unit reflecting symptoms, pathology, or dysfunction; an applied cybernetic approach recognizes that the world view and cultural attributes of the family counselor are interconnected with the client family. Family members interact and engage self-regulating and self-maintaining complementary roles. As such the family counselor, who is admitted into the family system on a temporary basis, plays a *complementary* role to the client family. In this role, the family counselor is positioned to gain some understanding of family relationship patterns that maintain a problem issue. More importantly, the novelty of the family counselor within the family system may serve to disrupt dysfunctional behavior patterns and help the family create more functional interactions.

The recursive relationship of the client family and family counselor continues throughout the therapeutic process and serves to construct a shared narrative about the issues that prompted the family to seek help. Equally important, this co-constructed narrative establishes a therapeutic context in which desired *change* takes place.

A culturally sensitive family counselor respects the client's right to *self identify*. In working with a client family, gaining an understanding of the importance the client places on a particular quality of characteristic is essential. For example, a family counselor might ask: "*What place does your Cuban heritage hold in your life?*" For some clients, national origin may be merely incidental. For others, such identity may be a central factor in their personal sense of self and identity.

Similarities and Differences in Intercultural Family Counseling

Acceptance of individual and group differences is an ethical responsibility of all counselors. Counselors may not discriminate on the basis of "*race, religion, creed, national origin, ethnicity, or sexual orientation*" (ACA, 2014) Although a moral and ethical value which respects diversity may seem self-evident, this concept may challenge and often compels an examination of the family counselor's personal beliefs and values, and how these may differ from those of the client.

All people possess a set of "core beliefs" – notions about "how things are," or at least "how things should be." Beginning in childhood, a client's "world view" is shaped by family cultural customs. Client views may be explicit or implicit and include such things as religious or spiritual beliefs and practices, philosophy, customs, marital and family roles and parenting practices – distinguishing behaviors that are "right" or "wrong," "proper" or "improper," and "acceptable" or "unacceptable." Often, such determinations are subjective, differing from culture to culture.

Depending upon the context, social and cultural rules may be codified in law or they may take the form of social customs. The consequences of violating cultural rules may result in deleterious consequences. In some instances, rule violations may result in imprisonment or even death (Canfield, 2018).

Recognizing the potential consequences of a client's choice, family counselors refrain from attempting to impose their own personal values upon their client. This ethical responsibility can present a challenge between the counselor's ethical responsibilities and the norms of the client's cultural community. The IAMFC code of ethics of the International Association of Marriage and Family Counselors (IAMFC) states: "*Marriage and family counselors do not engage in activities which violate the legal standards of their community*" (IAMFC, 2017). In supporting a client, the family counselor must ethically advocate for basic human rights without influencing or endorsing a client's choices that may conflict with the community cultural values in which the client physically or psychologically embedded. Examples include:

- The practice of "polygamy" which is considered culturally acceptable in some communities and has been widely practiced for millennia in many cultures. For example, although polygamous marriage is illegal in the United States and Mexico, it is none-the-less practiced informally in some communities in both countries. How could a family counselor explore this issue with a client family without condoning illegal behavior?
- In some cultures, gender roles are clearly defined, inflexible, and rigidly enforced by the community. How might a family counselor address the issue of gender rights and equality without violating cultural norms to the client's detriment?

In the USA and in many other Western countries, "same sex" marriage is legal. However, in some communities and regions of the world – such as east Africa and parts of the Middle East – same sex relationships violate community standards and laws and are a punishable criminal offense. In light of such considerations, how might a family counselor best support a client struggling with sexual orientation issues within the cultural context of a religious community or a country where homosexual behavior is unacceptable?

Co-constructing a Therapeutic Relationship

A key to a successful family counseling outcome is the formation of a collaborative relationship between the counselor and client. This requires completion of certain tasks, which are typically on-going and concurrent throughout the counseling process.

Task 1: Joining with the Client

An initial task, but one that is particularly important when the counselor and client are perceptually or demographically different in some cultural aspect

(Canfield, 2018). The opportunity to join with the client family begins with the initial in-session interactions between the client and the counselor. Immediate visual impressions are formed, and subsequently reinforced or modified by on-going interactions. A skilled counselor intentionally projects a visual impression (i.e. personal appearance, office décor, etc.) and engages in verbal and non-verbal behaviors interactions with therapeutic intent. Interactions with the client should not be left to chance, but should be deliberate for the purpose of constructing a therapeutic relationship.

Prior to delving into problem concerns, it is often useful to ask initial questions about the family's background or recent activities. Such questions might include:

- *"I would like to know some things about you, so that I might be of help. Can you tell me what each of you enjoy doing when you are not at work or school."*
- *"What do you like most about your family?"*
- *"Tell me about your most recent family event or outing."*
- *"What do you plan to do after you leave here today?"*

The family counselor may share appropriate personal disclosures to make a connection with the family or selected family members. An example would be: *"That's interesting that both of you like the music of Queen, I am a big fan too. What are your favorite Queen songs?"* Examples of *connecting disclosures* that serve to facilitate the "joining" process include:

- *"My Dad worked in the construction field too. I have always enjoyed doing things with my hands."*
- *"Like you, my wife is a 'stay-at-home' Mom. I think that is one of the most difficult jobs around!"*
- *"So, you like to duck hunt? I grew up in a family of avid hunters. What do you like most about hunting?"*

While such questions during the initial family counseling consultation session may appear unrelated to the purpose at hand, there is a therapeutic intent behind such exchanges. Questions and disclosures are a "socio-metric" technique for gathering information while simultaneously building a connection with the client based on shared interests or experiences. This disclosure joining technique is both initial and ongoing throughout the therapeutic process. The "casual" conversation is not random, but rather has a very specific intent.

Task 2: Alignment and Support of Family Members

Gaining and understanding the client's background will often reveal challenging experiences the family has faced. Experiences such as racial discrimination, can complicate the counseling relationship, particularly when the family counselor is of a different race. Some clients may not have personally suffered from discrimination in their own life, but may hold some degree of vicarious sensitivity resulting from discrimination inflicted upon family members or close friends. For clients whose families have experienced political oppression, expulsion, or genocide; cultural differences can be profound in terms of their sense of connection with the larger society. For example, a counselor who identifies as "Muslim" may find it challenging to overcome the negative perceptions some clients may hold of Muslims. Similarly, a young Black female counselor may find it challenging to effectively join with a middle-class White family, given possible assumptions of the part of the client or the family.

Cultural generalizations may be baseless and "unfair," but they can also be very real. It is essential that the family counselor address and strive to overcome perceived differences that may impede the counseling relationship. One strategy is for the counselor to directly address any possible concerns about cultural differences – "*when you walked into room and saw that I was a 55-year old White guy (or a 30-year old Black woman), what were your initial thoughts as to how we might be able to work together effectively?*" Following the client's response, a follow-up question might be: "*Have you ever had a similar experience, with people making assumptions about you, based on appearance* (or age, or gender, etc.)?"

Task 3: Establishing the Purpose and Goals of Family Counseling

It has long been recognized that clarifying the purpose and goal of family counseling is essential. It is often assumed that the primary goal for the client is ameliorating the presenting problem. While this may be the case, at times the client's goal may be unclear, or merely a symptom of a larger issue. It is common that various family members may hold different goals or outcomes in mind.

Establishing client goals requires exploration and research. Perhaps asking each family member in turn, the following questions may be useful in clarifying client expectations:

- "*Who would like to tell me what prompted you to come here today?*"
- "*What would you like to see come out of today's meeting?*"
- "*Tell me how I could be most helpful to you.*"
- "*How will you know when our work together is succeeding?*"

In furtherance of establishing the individual agendas and goals of family counseling, it is often useful at the end of the initial counseling session to assign an out-of-session task or assignment to the family. One such assignment is to ask each family member to separately to "*write down 'three or four things' that you would like to see different in your family. Give this some thought and bring your written list to our next session. For now, it is important that you keep this information to yourself – I ask that you not share your list with any other family member.*"

At the next session, the family counselor will review each list and engage the family in a discussion regarding shared and differing goals. This provides an initial set of possible goals for the family to discuss and prioritize.

Task 4: Defining and Clarifying the Role of the "Helper"

Counseling is a professional relationship in which a qualified counseling professional utilizes their knowledge and skills to assist the client in bringing about desired change. In a broad sense, the purpose of family counseling is to improve the quality of relationships and/or individual functioning within the context of interpersonal relationships. All people regardless of cultural identity encounter problems in living and problems endemic to the human condition. As such, every society recognizes individuals who possess knowledge and skill for helping others (Pesek, Helton, & Nair, 2006.) "Counseling" is only the most recent manifestation of this role, dating back thousands of years

Cultural views may create preconceived notions about the counseling process and the counselor. Among some clients it is assumed that the counselor is similar to a medical doctor treating an illness, holding a mistaken belief that the family counselor has the ability to "fix" a problem. The client presents the "problem" and the family counselor dispenses advice and directives, resulting in needed change ("*This is the problem, now tell us what to do, so this can be cured.*") Such a belief is understandable when the cultural expectations of a client view the role of the family counselor as the "expert." Such client families may prefer a more directive counseling approach and may not respond well to a more reflective counseling approach, and may even view the family counselor as lacking competence.

Since clients may hold an erroneous notion regarding the role of the counselor, it is essential that both client and counselor roles be discussed and agreed upon. A common parental request might be – "*I want you to work with my son and make him be a better student!*"

Contrary to the role of counselor as "expert," family counseling emphasizes the collaborative nature of the counseling relationship in which the client and family counselor work as a "team" to find solutions to concerns. The family counselor should take time during the initial session to discuss the collaborative nature of family counseling, while working within the family's cultural context. The family counselor should clearly convey that responsibility for bringing about desire change is primarily a responsibility of the family, with the active assistance of the counselor.

Task 5: Working with the Family to Accomplish Goals

A useful position for the family counselor to hold when working with any client – but particularly with a client who is culturally different from the family counselor – is one of "curiosity and interest." Since the status of the family counselor is already known to the client, adopting a *collaborative* rather than an *expert* posture allows the family counselor and client family to work together and appropriately define and divide tasks and responsibilities to ensure a successful outcome.

An understanding of the respective roles of the family counselor and family members is essential. This is particularly important when client cultural expectations may be based on erroneous assumptions regarding the scope and role of the family counselor in "fixing" the client's problem. Framing family counseling as a collaborative relationship between the counselor and client minimizes such misunderstandings. This strategy places the responsibility for change with family members. However, it also emphasizes the role of the family counselor as a knowledgeable resource – an ally who joins the family system and works as actively with family members to recognize dysfunctional behavioral patterns, problematic family roles and structure, and creating circumstances to bring about desired changes.

In bringing about desired change, it is the role of the family counselor to employ an array of intervention strategies to bring about desired changes. The specific theoretical orientation of the family counselor is less important than the capacity of the family counselor to join and work with the family in a collaborative manner.

Conclusions and Recommendations

There is no single theory or approach to counseling best suited to every client. The degree to which the family counselor can *join* with the client family and become part of a collaborative work effort is foundational to a successful therapeutic outcome. Effective intercultural family counseling requires that the counselor possess a basic knowledge and understanding of the client family's cultural orientation, and awareness of one's own cultural roots and influences.

An understanding of cultural differences, and utilization of a therapeutic approaches and techniques that present a "good fit" with the client provide the best opportunity for helping the client. As the saying goes, "one size does not fit all." While some aspects of family counseling are universal, in working with a specific family, the cultural dynamics often require a somewhat unique or specific approach. An approach that may work well with one client in one cultural context, may fall short with another client in another cultural context. As such, creativity and adaptability are essential. The following chapters in this book offer insight into working with specific relationship or family issues within a particular cultural context.

References

American Counseling Association. (2014). *Code of ethics and standards of practice*. Alexandria, VA: American Counseling Association.

Becvar, R., Canfield, B., & Becvar, D. (1997). *Group work: Cybernetic, constructivist, and social constructionist perspectives*. Denver, CO: Love Publishing.

Bitter, J. R. (2009). *Theory and practice of family therapy and counseling*. Belmont, CA: Brooks/Cole.
Canfield, B. (1999). *Relationship enrichment in counseling and human development*. Denver, CO: Love Publishing.
Canfield, B. (2018). *Family systems: Genograms and socio-metric assessment*. In C. Gill & R. Freund (Eds.), *Spirituality and religion in counseling: Competency based strategies for ethical practice*. New York: Taylor & Francis.
Canfield, B., & Locke, D. W. (1992). Professional identity and family therapy. In R. Smith & P. Stevens-Smith (Eds.), *Family counseling and therapy: Major issues and topics*. Greensboro, NC: Eric Caps.
International Association of Marriage and Family Counselors. (2017). *IAMFC code of ethics*. Alexandria, VA: IAMFC.
McGoldrick, M. (1998). *Re-visioning family therapy: Race, culture, and gender in clinical practice*. New York: Guilford.
Pesek, T., Helton, L., & Nair, M. (2006). *Healing across cultures: Learning from traditions. EcoHealth*, 3(2), 114–118.

Additional Resources

American Counseling Association – www.counseling.org.
American Association for Marriage and Family Therapy – www.aamft.org.
Association for Counselor Education and Supervision – www.acesonlinenet.
American Mental Health Counselors Association – www.amhca.org.
Association for Lesbian, Gay, Bi-sexual & Transgender Issues in Counseling – www.algbtic.org.
Association for Spiritual, Ethical, and Religious Values in Counseling – www.aservic.org.
Center for Multicultural Mental Health Research – www.multiculturalmentalhealth.org.
Center for Multilingual Multicultural Research – www.bcf.usc.edu.
Consortium for Multicultural Psychology Research – www.psychology.msu.edu/cmpr.
Ecohealth – www.springerlink.com.
International Association of Marriage and Family Counselors – www.iamfconline.org.

2

COUNSELING MUSLIM COUPLES AND FAMILIES IN THE UNITED STATES

Khalid A. Alfallatah

Introduction

As the counseling field engages in intercultural practice considerations, the need for researching different cultures increases. With more than 3 million Muslims living in the United States and about 1.5 billion others around the world the need for more research is increasing (Lipka, 2017). The Muslim population in the United States is growing and researchers in the mental health field are conducting more research related to this population (Ibrahim et al., 2015). This chapter provides an overview of Islamic family concepts along with a case study that will help readers better understand multiple ways of implementing clinical interventions when working with Muslim couples and families in the United States.

Many Muslim societies tend to be collectivistic and individualism is discouraged (Ali et al., 2004). The Quran repeatedly encourages showing respect to parents and discourages children from raising their voice on their parents. When major conflicts arise, practicing Muslim children who engage in arguments with their parents and raise their voice feel very guilty and find it very difficult to express their emotions to their parents.

Muslim clients will vary in the degree of their adherence to religious principles and practice. The variation of the degree of assimilation may create family conflicts. Recent immigrants may be considered more religious than individuals born in the United States (Ali et al., 2004). Conflicts between children and parents may arise regarding religious and spiritual Islamic issues. Therapists may need to assess the level of religiosity of both parents and their children to gather more data about the family.

Another aspect that should be noted by clinicians is that there are multiple factors that may prevent Muslim clients from seeking therapy. Research has revealed that one of the reasons Muslims hesitate to seek treatment is their fear of being stigmatized within the Muslim community. The fear of being stigmatized drives some clients to prefer using family/friends advice over seeking professional help.

Another barrier stems from the fear of being seen as inferior, or for looking ridiculous, or for being sensitive to their culture being criticized, which means not wanting to add to the negative stereotype about the Muslim culture if the problem becomes known to others outside of the culture. Furthermore, there is a gap in the literature in providing guidance for therapists about the best ways to approach Muslims living in the United States (Sauerheber, Nims, & Carter, 2013).

After understanding some of the barriers that can stop Muslim clients from seeking therapy, the understanding of the therapeutic relationship with Muslim women is essential. Alotaiby aimed to answer the following questions: What is the experience of marriage and family therapists with respect to issues of power inequality in the therapeutic relationship with Muslim women? And what do therapists do to make their practice applicable to work with Muslim women? The phenomenological study was conducted by interviewing 11 therapists that worked with Muslim couples and clients.

The results of this study revealed important themes (that are important for therapist to know) such as: (a) recognition of limitation and privilege; (b) accountability and accommodation.

The first theme described the recognition of limitations and privilege within the Muslim clients. An important sub-theme construct identified was accessibility. Therapists in this study shared that the accessibility factor appeared to have an influence on the therapeutic relationship. Accessibility was viewed differently by participants. For example, some therapists noted utilizing an interpreter to overcome the language barrier in cases where clients did not speak English. Others suggested that having a co-therapist from the same culture would support a stronger therapeutic relationship. It is important to note that some therapists might find it challenging to understand the Islamic culture and religion; however, a full understanding of the Islamic religion is not required for a successful therapeutic outcome.

The second sub-theme in this study was privilege, gender, and women's issues. In this category, therapists shared how their cultural backgrounds influenced their perception of clients throughout these experiences. Some therapists shared their feelings about being at a place of privilege in relation to race and socioeconomic status noting that they had to work on their own biases while building the therapeutic relationship. While it was hard for some therapists to relate to the difficulties some of the clients suffered, it was easier for others to relate to some aspects of the power and hierarchy paradigm, in which therapists could identify with what they shared with the clients through this experience.

Although therapists in this study noted that they were not experts in their clients' faith, nor did they have the experience some of the difficulties that their clients go through such as intense security checking while traveling or going through airports, some were able to connect with their clients by sharing some of their own experiences.

Gender is a very important factor to be aware of when interacting with clients of Islamic faith. Recognizing your own bias and perceptions about gender is of great importance to the therapeutic relationship with Muslim clients. The ability to relate to Muslim clients will help in forming a stronger relationship. Alotaiby noted that rather than seeing the client as only a Muslim woman, a therapist in her study, reflected on the humanity of the client, which had the greatest influence on the relationship with the client.

Another theme reveled in this study was accountability and accommodation. The main construct in this theme is adjustment to practice. What this sub-theme refers to is the ability to make certain adjustments when working with certain clients, for example, incorporating the cultures of the clients into the treatment. Some therapists reported they did more home visits, and ate with the clients, which it is not commonly something they would have done. Another therapist reported that she made assessments to incorporate the client's religion into the treatment.

Substance Abuse Interventions for Muslim Clients

Many studies had focused and researched the effectiveness of 12 steps programs on recovering addicts. The studies identified the effectiveness of multiple support groups such as A.A., Alanon, and N.A. and other support groups on individuals in recovery. Multiple factors such as family relationships and functioning in society were explored. However, very few studies have been conducted to explore the effectiveness of Milati Islami (MI), an Islamic-based 12-steps program for addicts. A thorough literature review will be conducted to explore the topic.

With the increase of substance use in the Muslim population in the USA, especially among the younger generation, looking at the effects of support groups such as Milati Islami becomes essential. Muslim addicts might feel more responsible when it comes to their relationship with their family. They might also feel responsible when it comes to their relationship with their higher power. These feelings could cause negativity and difficulty for addicts and their families. By understanding more about the 12-steps programs such as MI, researchers can help strengthen family relationships in addition to providing addicts with better conceptualization about their relationship with their higher power.

In a single month an estimated 20 million Americans aged 12 or older use an illegal drug as reported by the National Survey on Drug Use and Health (Alcohol and Drug Information). Less than 30% of all 2013 arrestees reported ever receiving any drug or substance abuse treatment. Among this population, more than 80% of arrestees noted that they have been arrested at least once prior to their current arrest (Alcohol and Drug Information). This cycle of drug use and arrest is a potential waste of human productivity and growth. The mental health field has to evaluate and advocate for a variety of support groups that can help client have different options when seeking treatment and support systems.

Family Relationship

There are no set rules that can measure the effects of having an alcoholic family member on adolescents in the family household. However, a significant improvement can be made when addicts and family members work on improving their self-concept.

A study aimed to investigate the associations between structural features of the self-concept and certain aspects of psychological adjustment among adolescents growing up in alcoholic families. In this study a sample of 60 adolescents from alcoholic families living in two large cities were examined. The three aspects of wealth, stability, and certainty of their self-concepts were evaluated using a set of questionnaires. The strongest association found in the study between richness of the self-concept and depression. That means that the more stable the self-concept, the lower the level of depression (Polak, Puttler, & Ilgen, 2012). In this research the emphasis on the self-concept helped improve depression. One of the main goals of support groups such as MI, A.A., and N.A. is to help members gain a better understanding of themselves (Ali, 2014). It remains essential to explore the effectiveness of the 12-steps programs on families with an addicted member.

The self-concept idea talked about in the previous research is not foreign to faith-based support system organizations. Research aimed at exploring the support system provided by faith-based organizations to families of clients undergoing substance use treatment explores the effects of such interventions. The research suggested that religious behaviors affected A.A. members, where belief did not (Kaskutas et al., 2003). Religious behaviors such as seeking family reconciliation and working on family issues can be very helpful for clients. Clients can be religiously motivated to work on family relationship issues. This suggests the importance of research in the literature about the effects of religious behavioral rituals on client's recovery. The research noted that one of the best methods of assessments when working with a substance abuser is to conduct a family assessment. It is recommended when working from a faith-based model to help families find hope and unity (Ali, 2014).

Relationship with Higher Power

The concept of higher power has its definition in the 12-steps program. The third step refers to the higher power as "God as we understand him" (Alcoholics

Anonymous, 2001). The literature addresses 12-steps programs and their diversity. Some programs are family-oriented and others are for specific age groups. There are also faith-based 12-steps programs such as Milati Islami (MI), which is Islamic based. There are some similarities and differences between MI and A.A. One major difference is that MI is based on an Islamic doctrine. A research aimed to explore the MI support group and compare it to the A.A. support group the research also addresses some Islamic concepts regarding addiction. All intoxicants are prohibited in Islam (Ali, 2014). Therefore a practicing Muslim client with substance use disorder may feel that their relationship with their higher power "Allah" is damaged. Therefore the existence of the MI support group can helps Muslim clients restore that relationship.

The 12 steps in MI are different but similar than the Alcoholic Anonymous 12 steps. The first step of A.A. is about admitting ones powerlessness over alcohol and that one's life had become unmanageable. In MI 12 steps it states that "We admitted that we were neglectful of our higher selves and that our lives have become unmanageable" (Ali, 2014). The MI version puts the responsibility on the person and used the word neglectful instead of powerless. In the Islamic faith, admitting neglecting can be a motivation for repentance.

In the second step, the A.A. 12-steps version noted that one came to believe that a power greater than oneself could restore their sanity. However, in the MI 12 steps it stated that "We came to believe that Allah could and would restore us to sanity" (Ali, 2014). Throughout the steps it can be noted that the MI steps are designed to address the specific needs of Muslim individuals with substance use problems.

More research needs to be conducted to examine the effectiveness of MI on clients that are practicing the Islamic faith and are substance users. This possible gap in the literature is worth of research and investigation as it can be considered an avenue that advocate and support Muslim clients.

Case Example

Jasmine is a 22-year-old Lebanese American Muslim female born in Orlando Florida. Her parents came to the United States from Lebanon and had her a year after their arrival. Jasmine is an only child. Her 45-year-old mother is a high school teacher at a local Islamic school. Her 50-year-old father is a physician at a local hospital. Jasmine described her family as being traditional and religious. She noted that she is a practicing Muslim and that she considers her faith to be important. Jasmine stated that she had multiple family conflicts in the past and that she is currently experiencing anxiety about wearing the hijab in public. She noted that with the increasing number of hate crime incidents against Muslims in the United States that she is considering to take off her headscarf "hijab."

Hijab is an Arabic word that means protection, cover, and barrier. Muslim women in America may at sometimes find it difficult to wear their Islamic hijab in public. Some Muslim women may decide to wear the hijab, niqab, or burqa, whereas others may decide to stop wearing them because of negative reactions and actions from others (Cole & Ahmadi, 2003). Those decisions of either wearing or taking off the hijab may lead to family conflicts within the Muslim family. Jasmine noted that her parents are opposed to her decision to stop wearing the hijab. She said that although she understands their point of view, she has concerns about her safety and discomfort.

Case Conceptualization, Clinical Assessments, and Interventions

Researchers to gather data about families over generations have long used genograms. Murray Bowen's family systems theory was one of the first theories of family systems functioning (Brown, 1999). Multigenerational transmission is an essential concept of the Bowen family systems theory. This concept explains how patterns and roles are passed from one generation to another. The theory not only focuses on family patterns as an evaluation process, but as a therapeutic intervention. When family members are able to learn more about the history of their family and times in which they got stuck, they are better able to look at and take responsibility for their own part in conflicts (Brown, 1999). Many researchers have developed and expanded on Bowen's work to be able to better understand the multigenerational transmission concept and other essential concept of the theory.

When conceptualizing Jasmine's case, the therapist must take into consideration multiple aspects. First, an examination of Jasmine's spiritual genogram is essential. The spiritual genogram is a tool developed to help clients gain different perspectives on ways in which their spiritual and religious history continues to affect their reactivity, reactions, and family processes (Frame, 2000).

The spiritual genogram can be used at any process of therapy and is used as an assessment strategy to gather data. After developing the appropriate client-counselor bond, trust, and getting the client's consent, the counselor would conduct the spiritual genogram. The counselor must make sure that using this tool is appropriate by assessing the presenting problem and the client's willingness to address religious and spiritual concerns (Frame, 2000).

The spiritual genogram involves four steps. Creation of the spiritual genogram, questions for future reflection, connection with one's family of origin, and integration into the global therapeutic endeavor are the four steps of the spiritual genogram (Frame, 2000). Understanding and implementing the four steps of the genogram are essential for acquiring a better understanding of the systemic perspective of the collected data.

The first step of creating the spiritual genogram is very important in that it helps in obtaining necessary information in the family's religious and spiritual history. In this stage, the therapist and client draw a three-generational family map including as much information as possible about family members. Important information such as significant events, births, marriages, divorces, and deaths are noted. Noting family member's religiosity, spirituality, and major significant religious and spiritual personal and community events is noted.

Events such as mosque vandalisms, threating letters to the congregation, changing in the racial/ethical or class composition of the congregation and/or other important events should be noted. Gathering information about client's perspective on family member's level of religiosity and spirituality is gathered. An example of an event could be a conflict between a mother and daughter when the daughter married outside her religion. Another example would be a conflict between a father and a son when the son changed his religious affiliation. The creation of the spiritual map/genogram is considered the first step of the assessment process.

The second step of the process is the questions for further client reflection. In this stage, the therapist asks questions with the intention of having the clients reflect on the role that religious/spiritual beliefs, experiences, rituals, and practices have on their presented issue. The questions aim to help clients externalize religious issues and reduce emotional reactivity in their relationships. In the next session, the therapist invites clients to share their insights about their responses and further reflect on the family dynamic in relation to religious and spiritual issues in the family (Frame, 2000). Some clients may not have all answers to those questions, which is a good place to proceed to step three, "connecting with one's family of origin."

In the third stage clients connect with their families of origin. This is an opportunity for clients to gain access to information from extended family members to clarify religious and spiritual events and elicit the meaning that family members attribute to those events (Frame, 2000). The additional information is added to the original genogram and the fourth stage is introduced.

In the fourth stage the therapist seeks to integrate the spiritual genogram created and the information gathered to process it with the family. In this process the family explores the effects of reflecting on their own past beliefs, experiences, and family-of-origin issues (Frame, 2000).

The process of exploring family's religious and spiritual journey helps the family reflect on issues that may contribute to the family's presenting problems. The application and use of the spiritual genogram will be integrated to address specific religious and spiritual Islamic concepts. Understanding essential issues about counseling families of Islamic faith can give a deeper understanding of the process of integrating the spiritual genogram when working with Muslim families.

Using the spiritual genogram with Muslim families would be helpful in gathering more data about the family and helping them reflect on their religious and spiritual presenting problem. Using the four stages of the spiritual genogram would help the therapist to make an assessment on family member's level of spirituality and religiosity.

The spiritual genogram may assist Muslim families to have a deeper understanding of the effects of different levels of religiosity and spirituality on conflicts in the family. The spiritual genogram can also be used to help Muslim families cope with stressors. Research aimed to investigate coping skills of Muslim women survivors of domestic violence. Researchers found that Muslim women who used spirituality were able to cope with ongoing domestic violence. The research indicated that religious coping mechanism included listening to Quran, prayer and meditation (Hassouneh-Phillips, 2001).

When integrating the spiritual genogram with Muslim families, it is important to take into consideration the diversity of the Muslim population. Muslim families may share a universal religion, but they exhibit diversity in relation to ethnic and racial history and heritage. In the third stage of the spiritual genogram where clients are connecting with families of origin, the intergenerational issues must be taken in consideration. The therapist would help clients reflect on how religious values and cultural norms were and are talked about (Sauerheber, Nims, & Carter, 2013).

Generational patterns can help families gain more awareness of their degree of differentiation and their level of emotional separation from their family of origin (Kerr & Bowen, 1988). The religious, spiritual,l and cultural values passed down from one generation to the other affects the development of a differentiated person within a family system (Bartle-Haring, Glebova, & Meyer, 2007). Using this process with Muslim families can help clients get a better understanding of each member's contribution to the presenting problem.

When counseling Muslim families, a good assessment of their level of religious, spiritual, and cultural values is essential. The assessment along with counseling skills and techniques creates an appropriate environment to foster a healthy therapeutic process.

The use of the spiritual genogram and the process of integrating that tool in relation to conflicts among Muslims facing social injustice, stereotyping and family conflicts can be beneficial in helping those families move forward. The need of an academic discussion about whether the spiritual genogram can work across cultures and believes is a good area of future research. Researching whether or not family levels of spirituality or religiosity may affect or play a role in hindering or expediting the therapeutic outcome is recommended. With the rising number of Muslims in the USA and worldwide, the need to explore different interventions and the implications of them becomes more prevalent to the counseling field.

Conclusions and Recommendations

Counseling Muslim couples and families in the USA is an area that needs to be explored. Researchers focused on multiple factors which seem to help clinicians gain a better understanding and better results with their Muslim clients.

Understanding that Muslim clients will vary in the degree of their adherence to religious principles and practice will help clinicians in planning appropriate interventions and create treatment plans collaboratively with their clients.

In addition to that, it is important that clinicians are aware of their own biases and perceptions about Muslim clients. Researchers revealed that some barriers that can stop Muslim clients from seeking professional help stem from the fear of being seen as inferior or for being sensitive to their culture being criticized, which means not wanting to add to the negative stereotype about the Muslim culture if the problem becomes known to others outside of the culture. With all the stereotypes about Muslims in the media and more, Muslim clients are very sensitive to any bias that might be presented by therapists which could jeopardous the therapeutic relationship.

Religion is often an integral part of Muslim clients and needs to be addressed by the multiculturally aware counselor. This will help therapists gain better understanding of how clients perceive themselves, others, and the world. That will also help guide therapeutic interventions. An example of that would be to explore if your client feels that joining the Milati Islami instead of a general 12-step programs is a better option for them.

It is also important to consider that for many Muslims, following their parents' wishes is considered to be a very important good faith indicator. Therefore, in situations where the child has a fundamental difference in opinion with their parents, that feeling of guilt and shame may be present. The therapist must be culturally competent and take into consideration that aspect in treatment planning and in therapy. Asking questions and being client-oriented would be the best way to have a successful therapeutic outcome.

References

Alcoholics Anonymous. (2001). *Alcoholics Anonymous* (4th ed.). New York: A.A. World Services.

Alcohol and Drug Information. (n.d.). Retrieved July 13, 2018, from https://ncadd.org/for-the-media/alcohol-a-drug-information.

Ali, M. (2014). Perspectives on drug addiction in Islamic history and theology. *Religions*, 5 (3), 912–928. doi:10.3390/rel5030912.

Ali, S. R., Liu, W. M., & Humedian, M. (2004). Islam 101: Understanding the religion and therapy implications. *Professional Psychology: Research and Practice, 35*(6), 635–642. doi:10.1037/0735-7028.35.6.635.

Bartle-Haring, S., Glebova, T., & Meyer, K. (2007). Premature termination in marriage and family therapy within a Bowenian perspective. *The American Journal of Family Therapy*, 35, 53–68.

Brown, J. (1999). Bowen family systems theory and practice: Illustration and critique. *Australian and New Zealand Journal of Family Therapy, 20*(2), 94–103. doi:10.1002/j.1467-8438.1999.tb00363.x.

Chamberlin, J. (2004, August 2). More Americans are seeking mental health treatment. Retrieved June 10, 2018 from www.apa.org/monitor/julaug04/survey.aspx.

Cole, D., & Ahmadi, S. (2003). Perspectives and experiences of Muslim women who veil on college campuses. *Journal of College Student Development*, 44, 47–66.

Frame, M. W. (2000). The spiritual genogram in family therapy. *Journal of Marital & Family Therapy*, 26(2), 211–216.

Hassouneh-Phillips, D. (2001). Polygamy and wife abuse: A qualitative study of Muslim women in America. *Journal of Mental Health in Nursing*, 22, 735–748.

Ibrahim, N., Kamsani, S. R., & Champe, J. (2015). Understanding the Islamic concept of Usrah and its application to group work. *Journal for Specialists in Group Work, 40*(2), 163–186. doi:10.1080/01933922.2015.1017067.

Kaskutas, L. A., Turk, N., Bond, J., & Weisner, C. (2003). The role of religion, spirituality and Alcoholics Anonymous in sustained sobriety. *Alcoholism Treatment Quarterly*, 21(1), 1–16. doi:10.1300/J020v21n01_01.

Kerr, M. E., & Bowen, M. (1988). *Family evaluation: An approach based on Bowen theory*. New York: W. W. Norton & Company.

Lipka, M. (2017, June 8). Muslims and Islam: Key findings in the U.S. and around the world. Retrieved June 15, 2017, from www.pewresearch.org/.

Polak, K. A., Puttler, L. I., & Ilgen, M. A. (2012). The relationship between structural aspects of self-concept and psychosocial adjustment in adolescents from alcoholic families. *Substance Use & Misuse, 47*(7), 827–836. doi:10.3109/10826084.2012.672536.

Sauerheber, J. D., Nims, D., & Carter, D. J. (2013). Counseling Muslim couples from a Bowen family systems perspective. *The Family Journal, 22*(2), 231–239. doi:10.1177/1066480713514937.

3

FAMILY COUNSELING IN UGANDA

Daniel Williamson and Jennifer Williamson

Introduction

Marriage and Family Counseling in Uganda is a multicultural experience even for native Ugandans. Uganda includes 17 distinct ethnic tribes with 45 individual languages. Although most counselor training is conducted in English, when counseling, many clients are more comfortable expressing themselves in their native tongues, so it is desirable to match counselors with clients' language. Feelings are not openly expressed in many Ugandan families and tribes, and emotions are often hidden. Counselors in Uganda must be sensitive to the cultural heritage of all family members and take an approach that embraces both traditional and modern beliefs (Senyonyi, Ochieng, & Sells, 2012). There is great pride in preserving traditions, social obligations, appropriate behaviors, and preserving individual dignity. It is imperative to recognize that the issues of Uganda are best conceptualized, understood, and addressed in most situations from the unique perspectives of Ugandans. Advocates can provide supports and seek to understand, but it is important that a position of support and cross-cultural collaboration be addressed rather than one of imperialism or top-down education.

Traditionally, when problems arise within the families, uncles and aunts engage performing as indigenous family therapists. This pattern continues to prevail throughout rural Africa communities, particularly when siblings live close together. Siblings often see their nieces and nephews as their own children and feel obligated and free to intervene in family issues. In some areas, it is acceptable for village members to intervene in child-rearing or to discipline a child. However, there has been a push for urbanization and with it a fragmentation of the traditional communal family structures of tribal life (Nwoye, 2006), thus creating an even larger need for professional counseling.

Ugandan Family Structures

In the rural village of Bulike, Uganda, traditionally marriage is polygamistic. Men can marry multiple wives throughout life, and a man's value is measured by the number of children he fathers. Marriages are often arranged with an exchange of property from the groom to the bride's father. Multiple wives might be seen as a sign of wealth or prosperity. The conversion from traditional faith practices to Christianity has created an opportunity for individuals to question marital practices in ways that have not previously been allowed. As girls gain more education and make greater contributions to family (of origin) income, daughters are able to delay marriage and have a greater voice in spousal selection (Kaluya, 2014). It is important to define and understand the family unit in Uganda as defined by the couple or family. In finding ways to better understand family dynamics and structure, modified genograms can help identify relational struggles, estrangement, discord, abuse, and conversely, sources of support, and strong familial bonds.

Child-Rearing

In many parts of Western culture, children are typically raised by their own parents and immediate family. However, in Uganda, there is often a communal nature to child-rearing and in understanding *Who raised you?* The exploration of "mothering" in parts of Africa might require at least two questions: *Who bore you?* and *Who reared you?* (Isiugo-Abanihe, 1985). Many times, children can be placed in the care of a benevolent godparent for a period of time without legal intervention. In areas where child fostering is prevalent, family systems might be more complex than Western systems and require greater exploration on part of the counselor.

Shame, Ostracism, and the Importance of Empathy

Shame and ostracism are two common methods of social punishment in Ugandan families and can be psychologically damaging to individuals and families especially when circumstances are beyond their control (Kaluya, 2014). Brown (2007) identified that the single strongest antidote for shame is empathy and counselor approaching clients with Roger's core conditions of genuineness, empathy, and unconditional positive regard in mind, will likely have more success connecting with clients and avoiding the risk of shame dominating the counseling experience (Rogers, 1942). Shame and ostracism are especially difficult for people of Uganda as their tribal culture is intensely relational and there is great fear of being alone. "Shame is about the fear of disconnection" (Brown, 2007, p. 27) and for rural Ugandan families, connection is not only psychologically necessary but a key element for survival (Kaluya, 2014).

Sexual Violence

Sexual violence against women has been an issue that has plagued both rural and urban areas of Uganda. Kaluya (2014) identified that "while the majority of educated Ugandans agree that rape is wrong and should be punishable to the person doing it, in Uganda there are no laws that implicate married couple or spouses who choose to force themselves onto the married partner. Kaluya also suggested that "The absence of laws coupled with the cultural belief that women have no say when it comes to sexual issues leads to many women being forced into sex and yet have no one to report to this gross violence and abuse" [*sic*] (p. 7). Traditionally, women and girls sought help within the family from mothers, aunties, and sisters. The prevailing sentiment was to maintain silence as it was shameful to speak of such events. Additionally, it was very common for daughters to be treated as chattel and given to men temporarily or for marriage to settle a debt. Addressing these issues can be quite challenging because of the sensitive nature of the issue. Educating people and creating an awareness of the nature of the problem was the first step in talking about abuse, neglect, and violence. As men are often see as more credible, it is important that they introduce the concern for discussion. It is, however, important for all to bring the discussion to both women and younger girls of the village. feedback has suggested that creating an awareness about this type of abuse is somewhat effective in current marriages and families; however, it will be most effective by changing the ideas that are passed on to children (UCSS, 2015).

Widows and Orphans

An unfortunate characteristic of having a tightly connected family is that sometimes widows and orphans do not fit easily within a social structure. As unconnected individuals, they have lost their advocates and social power leaving them at risk for displacement, abuse, and neglect. In some families, these individuals are easily folded into extended families especially when affection exists for the parent who passed. However, in other circumstances, they are displaced or abandoned (UCSS, 2015).

Domestic Violence

Domestic Violence including sexual assault continues to be an issue in Uganda in both urban and rural areas. Unicef (2000) reported that 41% of women surveyed reported having been beaten by their husbands, and 41% of men report having beaten their wives. In rural areas, it is sometimes an expectation that physical violence is a normal part of married life. Additionally, as rape is also widespread and often misunderstood within the context of the marital relationship, Uganda Counseling and Support Services (2015) has instituted education programs for community outreach that educate men, utilizing male instructors, as to what constitutes rape, even within the context of a marriage. Similarly, male and female Ugandan outreach workers educate women on what is appropriate and not appropriate. Although many women continue to tolerate rape and domestic violence, especially within the bounds of marriage, there has been progress in prevention efforts. One of the hypotheses for the UCSS program is that women will pass this knowledge on to their sons and daughters which will eventually break the cycle of domestic, interpersonal violence. In addition to domestic violence and rape prevention education, psychoeducation addressing parenting, well-couples, and marital enrichment have been used to help relieve relational strain between couples and within families. This is a complex effort as many marriages continue to be polygamous in nature with one man and multiple wives and many children. Wolff, Blanc, and Gage (2000) concluded that "Women's ability to negotiate the timing and conditions of sex with their partners is central to their ability to control a variety of reproductive health outcomes" (p. 303). They also recognized that the "sexual double standards constrain women's sexual authority within unions as well as outside of them" (p. 305). Women's sexual power is often officially or unofficially left under their husband's control. Common early sexual socialization practices within the community dictate that women are not to deny their husband of sex when expected. This is especially true in areas where polygamy is still employed. Wolff, Blanc, and Gage (2000) speculated that senior wives and brides in monogamous unions are able to retain more power within their relationship.

The Idea of Marital Partnerships and Parenting

Traditionally, men in some rural Ugandan villages have identified three main roles they play in family life: fathering children, building a house or houses, and brewing alcohol. Counseling and psychoeducational programs that help men recognize the importance of their role in the family can be increasingly effective in helping them find additional ways to contribute to the welfare of the family. Warrington (2013) found that parental involvement, especially with fathers, had the ability to increase self-esteem and promote academic and career success in daughters. A major extrinsic factor was also the role of biological parents and networks of people who served as surrogate parents and mentors. Many couples have identified the desire to learn more about counseling and psychoeducational opportunities to enhance their marriage and family lives. Mujuzi (2010) identified that the Odozi Commission concluded on women's rights that "Ugandans had great expectations that the equality of women with men would be guaranteed in all aspects of life 'in the new Constitution and the new society governed by it.'" The commission documented the importance the Ugandan people place on family and expressed concerns with the right to marry and form families when it is "interfered with by tribal customs on grounds of race, tribe, creed or socioeconomic status and that the rights of both spouses as to marriage, during marriage and at its dissolution are not recognized nor respected" [*sic*] (417–418).

Gottman (Gottman & Silver, 1999) proposed the elimination of four elements from all marriages. He identified them as the four horsemen: criticism, contempt, defensiveness, and stonewalling. Gottman explained that complaining is good as it allows each member of the relationship to clearly articulate his or her feelings. Complaining is most effective with the use of *I* statements. *I hate it when there are so many clothes to wash* or *I wish I had something to eat when I arrive home.* In complaining, the focus is not on the fault of either spouse, but rather upon the circumstances.

Criticism involves attacking someone's personality or character. Examples would involve *You always* … or *You never.* Contempt is a more severe form of criticism and involves attacking the partner's sense of self-worth or attempting to psychologically abuse or mistreat him or her. This can include hostile humor, insults, and name calling, mockery, or derogatory body language (facial expressions, eye rolling, or sneering.) Defensiveness includes denying responsibility, making excuses, or cross complaining. Defensiveness tends to escalate conflicts rather than deescalating them. Stonewalling is the emotional removal of oneself from a situation. The *stonewaller* becomes a *stone wall.* The stonewaller claims to remain neutral. Gottman indicated that men are more likely to stonewall as they are more easily overwhelmed by marital conflict than women. Gottman also encourages couples to allow their partners to influence them, to work toward successful repair attempts in conflicts, and to create shared stories that are positive (Gottman & Silver, 1999).

Couples counseling can help couples focus on the relationship rather than on power, control, or blame. The counseling process can help couples to move toward a mutually empathic connection with each other while helping maintain a more balanced and egalitarian relational dynamic. Patience, cooperation, and kindness should be fostered as the possibility of competition may emerge in polygamous situations. Issues of power should be identified and appropriately addressed in a culturally humble manner as second and subsequent wives, young wives, and very old wives might not have the same power as primary wives, educated wives, and wives from families with resources. As the couple can foster a "we-ness" they can share in the concern while alleviating guilt, shame, and blame.

Infertility

Because of strong familial ties, both infertility and infant mortality are deeply difficult personal tragedies. While infertility affects people worldwide, in Uganda, women often bare the blame when concerns of infertility arise. The World Health Organization (2010) reported that more than 186 million ever-married women maintain a "child-wish," translating to one in every four couples in the world. In Uganda, women are often not well accepted by society if they do not have a child. Children are treasured and are used as a measurement for assessing the success of a marriage (Nwoye, 2006). Although male infertility has been found to be the cause in many cases, the social burden often falls to women. This is exacerbated by the social competition in a polygamistic marriage and the fear of not being cared for in old age. Gibson and Myers (2000) indicated that the existing research identifies that woman sharing their stories, in relationship both with others and with partners, is a major tool for coping. Providing counseling services for couples where the conversation can occur in a safe space is an essential to establishing trust and confidence with the client. Gibson and Myers (2000) proposed using a relational model approach so that couples can benefit even when only one partner is able or willing to attend. The goal is to foster empathy and mutuality as both are necessary for growth (Jordan, 1997).

Revisiting Shame within the Context of Childbearing

Shame is a critical factor to consider as the ability to bear children is a critical life task in Ugandan marriages. As mentioned earlier, empathy is crucial to the elimination of shame (Brown, 2007). Group counseling for women experiencing infertility might be an approach where counselors can offer an alternative system of support so that other women with similar experiences can provide a normalizing effect as it relates to the struggle, potentially alleviating shame and guilt, while helping women cope with feelings of isolation and stigmatization. Counselors should attend to similarities that emerge in the group process and help women make connections in similarity of experience. Individual healing and coping can have positive effects on the marriage. As Siegel (1996) reported, "Here in Africa, the family is first. This will never change" (p. 221).

HIV Prevention, Coping, and Caregiving

Much has been written on the topic of Africa and the spread of HIV. This chapter has not addressed it as HIV is often viewed by many as an individual issue; however, coping, prevention, and caregiving of the disease are also family issues. This is especially complicated when exploring the strain experienced by family members and caregivers for those who may be suffering its effects. Counselors typically address HIV in a variety of ways. The most common are education and prevention, coping, and caregiving. Prevention is tricky as it is frequently viewed as unpopular. It asks for individuals and couples to have intentional conversations, engage in prophylactic measures, and refrain from risky behaviors. This often factors into the discussions of sexual and relational power discussed earlier in the chapter. Additionally, tradition plays a part in this dilemma. Albert, Akol, L'Engle, Tolley, Ramirez, Opio, Tumwesigye, Neema, and Baine (2011) identified that male circumcision has been found to reduce the sexual transmission of HIV from women to men. They also identify the World Health Organization's recommendation for medical male circumcision in areas of Africa where males are not widely circumcised and HIV rates are high; however, they discuss that in some African regions the acceptance of these practices are influenced by "social, cultural, and religious beliefs" (p. 1578).

Caregiving is a large concern with the presence of HIV in Uganda. Mugisha, Scholten, Owilla, Naidoo, Seeley, Chatterji, Kowal, and Boerma (2013) identified that "Older caregivers have major caregiving responsibilities in countries severely affected by the HIV epidemic" (p. 1341). They contended that in many cases a greater burden of caregiving is accompanied by weakened reciprocal care because of mortality of adult children. Not having children to care for their aging parents may impact the mental and physical health of older caregivers. Among the female caregivers, 85% have been identified as widows. Interestingly, most identified an enhanced sense of purpose, usefulness, and accomplishment in their caregiving roles. The most common difficulty in caregiving was a lack of energy and ability to take care of their own personal health issues. Counseling and psychoeducation focused on caregiver support will likely serve the people of Uganda well. For those who identify as being the only adults in the home, group counseling might help normalize their experience while developing coping strategies for dealing with isolation. As collectivism and relational concerns are a strong element associated with Uganda's culture, group counseling will also help caregivers develop support networks outside of the family of origin (UCSS, 2017).

Career Counseling

As identified earlier in the chapter, education and earning potential can serve to protect young females from being subjected to forced sexual encounters including early arranged marriage. Career counseling groups can be utilized as a tool for helping these women identify vocational resources and build vocational skills. Through skill development and education young girls can become economic contributors to the family and secure a choice in whom and when she marries. Women and girls are taught how to sew, raise pigs and chickens, grow agriculture, and make crafts for sale. This money can be used toward school fees or contributed to the family which makes it economically possible and beneficial for families to keep daughters longer within the family prior to marriage.

Narrative Therapy

The collectivistic and social nature of Ugandan culture lends itself well to therapeutic techniques and orientations that utilize those characteristic elements. Narrative Therapy is one of those unique approaches that embraces family and individual narratives. The role of stories that already exists in many tribes, can be used to help individuals within the family and couples to *re-story* their lives. This technique provides a powerful means for couples and families to co-create a shared narrative. Families can use narrative therapy to rewrite difficult stories and to arrive at a new meaning. Creating a shared story can help a family to have the courage to move forward through difficulties and come together. White and Epston (1990) posit "As discussed, in a therapy of oral tradition, the reauthoring of lives and relationships is achieved primarily, although not exclusively, through a process of questioning" (p. 17). They go on to explain "the re-storying of experience necessitates the active involvement of persons in the reorganization of their experiences" (p. 18).

Although an oral tradition approach fits well in Uganda, the idea of telling a story that is individual and that divulges personal secrets and pain might be radical from a cultural standpoint. The idea of identifying a villain in this narrative might also be seen as betrayal as many times it is a family member or close family friend who serves as perpetrator in the narrative; however, it is important that counselors recognize the therapeutic possibilities when helping clients to find their story, tell their story, and potentially rewrite the ending of their story. There is power in finding one's voice even when it is only used in private. Nwoye (2006) identifies that listening to a client's story is the best way to understand its genealogy. Bruner (1986) stresses that "Narrative structures organize and give meaning to experience, but there always feelings and lived experience not fully encompassed by the dominant story" (p. 143). Counselors have the opportunity to help clients to honor the struggle and to recognize the elements that can be controlled.

Importance should also be placed upon externalizing the problem. Too often, individuals feel as though they are a mistake rather than they have made a mistake or have been a victim. Externalizing is an approach to therapy that encourages persons to objectify and, at times, to personify the problems that they experience as oppressive. Therapists can guide couples in families toward externalizing the problem by utilizing relative influence questions. Relative influence questioning comprises two sets of questions: mapping the influence of the problem and mapping the influence of the person. Through externalization, unproductive conflicts can be decreased, a sense of failure can be undermined or eliminated, new possibilities can be opened up, and the way can be paved for persons to cooperate with each other. Finding ways to separate themselves and their relationships from the problem opens up the possibilities for them to describe themselves, each other, and their relationships from a new, nonproblem-saturated perspective, it enables the development of an alternative story, one that may be more attractive to family life (White & Epston, 1990).

Like narrative therapy, solution-focused brief therapy moves the client from a problem saturated narrative to a focus on solutions. This approach assists clients in focusing on the situations over which they have control. In solution-focused brief therapy there are a series of questions that can be employed by therapists: the exception finding question, the miracle question, the first sign question, and the scaling question (Berg, 1994).

Adlerian Counseling

Nwoye (2006) calls for the implementation of multicultural healing methods that work well with the globalized nature of the contemporary world. Adlerian therapy has been well received in Uganda as it is culturally sensitive, egalitarian, teleological, and phenomenological. Dreikurs (1967) identified four Adlerian phases of therapy: establishing a therapeutic relationship, interpretation, insight, and reeducation. All good therapeutic relationships emphasize the importance of the therapeutic alliance. Clients must feel comfortable and confident in this relationship to progress. During the interpretation phase, it is crucial that the clients' readiness for change is assessed. Prior to achieving insight, clients are not always aware that their lifestyles and private logic are interfering with their ability to make meaningful change. Clients might be weighing advantages and disadvantages of change. The counselor must be aware of the clients' readiness for change as action-oriented interventions in the therapeutic process might not be prudent. It is imperative that counselors are utilizing instruments and ideas that are relevant and sensitive to the culture. As therapists observe client change, it is imperative to recognize that readiness for change does not reside exclusively with the client; however, it is important to explore the readiness for change on the individual level, the family systems level, and even at times the cultural level. Although an individual might be open to change, there might be substantial reasons why he or she might hesitate. This might be especially true when working with clients in collectivistic cultures like Uganda.

As clients develop insight individuals may start and stop behavioral change. Encouragement and fostering an encouraging environment are crucial to the therapeutic process. Counselors should tap into the clients' creative process, helping the client to have the courage to be imperfect. Clients demonstrate overt behavioral, experimental, and environmental changes when addressing problems. Counselors also explore the basic needs of each member of the familial unit known as the Crucial Cs: count, connection, capable, and courage. Each member of a family needs to feel that he or she matters within the family (count), to feel as a part of the group (connection), to feel able to make a contribution (capable), and the ability to try even when uncertain (courage) (Bettner & Lew, 1989). In a collectivistic culture characteristic of Uganda, ensuring all members of a family or community find ways to meet theirs and others' Crucial Cs can serve as a primary therapeutic goal.

Satirian Counseling

Both Satir and Adler recognized the importance of the *family of origin* when working with families and couples. Adlerians employ the exploration of family constellation, early recollections, birth order, and lifestyle analysis when trying to understand the rules for living that individuals bring to the family dynamic. Satir explored the intrapsychic systemic model often conceptualized as an iceberg. On the surface individuals identify behaviors that are troublesome; however, beneath the surface are feelings, feelings about feelings, perceptions, expectations, yearnings, and a sense of self that exists and influences behaviors. It is important for the therapist to explore those feelings and ideas that lurk below the surface. Additionally, in family therapy, Satir emphasized the role of the therapist. She identified four meta-goals for change: raising the self-esteem of the client, helping the client to be their own choice-maker, helping the client to be more responsible, and helping the client to be more congruent. In family therapy, the family unit serves as the client. When utilizing Satir's model with families it is important to remember eight core beliefs:

1. There is a strong belief that change is always possible, even if change can only take place inside of the person. These changes might include feelings, perceptions, and expectations.
2. Therapy sessions need to be experiential in order to bring about second level change. This involves a change in being, not only in doing or feeling.
3. The problem is not the problem; coping is the problem. Therefore, therapy focuses on improving one's coping instead of just solving one's problems.
4. Feelings belong to us and, therefore, we can learn to change them, manage them, and enjoy them.
5. Therapy sets positively directional goals and resolves the impact of negative experiences.
6. Therapy is systemic, both intrapsychically and interactively.
7. People have the resources they need to cope and grow. Therapy is one vehicle to harness these resources to help people change.
8. Most people choose familiarity over the discomfort (Banmen, 2002, p. 8).

These core beliefs can be utilized to direct the therapeutic process or as tools in psychoeducation.

Community Action and Advocacy

In developing nations, it is important to recognize the need for community action, education, and advocacy when considering interventions that will have a lasting impact on the quality of life for couples and families. The common factors research indicates that extra-therapeutic factors account for 40% of improvements in successful outcomes. The therapeutic relationship accounts for 30%; placebo, hope, and expectancy account for 15%, and 15% is accounted for by specific models and techniques (Hubble, Duncan, & Miller, 1999). Keeping this in mind, a holistic approach to wellness should be considered that recognizes Maslow's Hierarchy of Needs where individuals will work toward satisfying basic physical needs prior to considering working toward more abstract psychological concerns

(Kaluya, 2014; Berk, 2018; Maslow, 1943). Programs that pair physical and psychological services might be considered. Programs seem to be most well received when individuals deeply tied to the communities are instrumental to the implementation and design. Additionally, Senyonyi, Ochieng, and Sells (2012) envisioned the integration of technology as a means of serving clients across Uganda. They recognized the importance of professional development training that embraces both traditional and modern cultural practices. Kaluya (2014) recommended the training of indigenous leaders and village elders as mental health facilitators. Through the use of programs like that developed by NBCC-I, more Ugandans can have access to mental health first aid (NBCC-I, 2012). This program sought to train trusted members of the community to identify those who might be experiencing difficulty and help connect them with mental health providers. As there is a scarcity of mental health resources throughout the rural community, it became increasingly important to have trusted members who could serve as a first contact for seeking help.

Case Examples

Joe and his wife, Mary, came to counseling because of difficulties in their marriage. Joe is unhappy because Mary has been angry with him, and he feels she has been neglecting him. Mary feels that Joe has been cruel because he has been yelling when he is at home, spending the family money, and staying away from home. As a result, Mary is having a hard time covering the children's school fees. The children miss him when he is away, especially his favorite daughter, Iris.

Joe and Mary seem to be experiencing very common difficulties. The therapist might employ an Adlerian approach emphasizing the value of social interest. In coaching them in *ways of caring*, the counselor might explain the necessity of sustenance caring, intentional caring, and reverential caring. Through the lens of caring, the therapist might explore the needs each of them identify and how they might meet those needs for each other. Reframing complaints from negative complaints to ways of caring can help couples to foster empathy, avoid blame, and build social interest. This new vocabulary can help to foster social interest and facilitate change. The therapist should approach this within the Adlerian phases of therapy and readiness for change. The counselor might explore the readiness for change at the individual level, the family systems level, and the cultural level.

The therapeutic process would begin by establishing the appropriate relationship with the clients and assessing their strengths and readiness for change. Through the lens of caring, the counselor can help clients to identify what they each need and what they can provide to their partner. It is important that the therapist identify the rate of change the clients both desire and can tolerate for success to occur.

Milton is a 30-year old community leader from a rural village. He has received some education, and he is curious about the idea of counseling and seeks help from a counselor in a medical clinic in his area. He would like to go to counseling with his wife, Kaikara, to explore ways of parenting their children. They have many fights concerning this issue. His wife is very traditional, but through his education, he is beginning to question some of the traditional approaches to child-rearing. Because he received some medical training, he is not sure about his son's participation in the community's circumcision ritual, and he is concerned about the possibility of HIV infection. His wife believes that this is an important part of growing up, and she wants her son to participate so that he is respected in the village and so he will remain close to her and take care of her when she is old. Additionally, they disagree on how to punish their younger children.

The counselor might employ a Satirian approach by exploring the intrapsychic systemic model (the iceberg). The counselor might explore beneath the surface to identify feelings, feelings about feelings, perceptions, expectations, yearnings, and a sense of self that exist and influence behaviors. Milton and Kaikara might possess strong feelings about traditions, and it would be important for the counselor to help them to explore these feelings and perceptions for themselves as well as for each other. It might also be important to help the couple identify what rules are negotiable and which are not. Once the couple understands the situation in greater depth, it might be easier to proceed. Additionally, the counselor might utilize Gottman's four horsemen technique to teach Milton and Kaikara how to discuss these issues fairly without the toxic damage that these four components can bring. Counselors might be aware of the Adlerian phases of therapy as they progress with Milton and Kaikara.

Dembe is an 11-year old girl whose father is exploring potential husbands because he has too many children to feed. Dembe is spirited and independent, willing to work hard, enjoys school and learning, and wants to help her family. Dembe has been assaulted by a man in the village, but she has not shared this with her family as she is concerned about ostracism, and she is told by aunties about things that are not discussed. Dembe earns very good grades, and her teacher is encouraging her to stay in school. She is frightened that she will be forced to leave school to get married. Her father has 12 other children, and Dembe is the oldest girl. Her mother is her father's second wife and possesses less influence with her husband. She sometimes cries when she sees the man who hurt her and tries very hard to push it out of her mind. She feels that it would be helpful if she had someone to talk to about these issues.

Dembe's counselor might consider two different approaches with her. First, there is a practical concern of money. Through career counseling and training, Dembe might be able to learn a skill that can contribute to her family's income which might allow them to give her some say in who and when she will marry. This might empower Dembe within the family system, and it might also impact her self-image. Secondly, the counselor should address the trauma that Dembe has endured. Although Dembe is not exhibiting negative behaviors or external difficulties, it might be very important to offer a safe place for her to talk about what has happened to her and how the event influences her self-image. Through employing a narrative approach, the counselor can help Dembe recognize that this is not her fault, and it is ok to talk about it. The counselor can help her to identify ways of coping with additional symptoms that she might not have identified prior to coming to counseling, and to externalize what has happened from who she is. Finally, through counseling, Dembe can be offered an opportunity to re-define the event as a past event that happened while allowing her to re-story the meaning that she gives to the circumstance, encouraging her to change her identity from that of victim to survivor. Counseling can provide both practical skills and instruction as well as a safe space where clients can process the difficulties in their lives.

References

Albert, L. M., Akol, A., L'Engle, K., Tolley, E. E., Ramirez, C. B., Opio, A., Tumwesigye, N. M., Thomsen, S., Neema, S., & Baine, S. O. (2011). Acceptability of male circumcision for prevention of HIV infection among men and women in Uganda. *AIDS Care*, 23(12), 1578–1585. doi:10.1080/09540121.2011.579939.

Banmen, J. (2002). The Satir model: Yesterday and today. *Contemporary Family Therapy*, 24, 7–22. doi:10.1023/A:1014365304082.

Berg, I. K. (1994). *Family-based services: A solution-focused approach*. New York: W. W. Norton & Company.

Berk, L. E. (2018). *Development through the lifespan* (7th ed.). Boston, MA: Pearson Publishing.

Bettner, B. L., & Lew, A. (1989). *Raising kids who can*. Newton Centre, MA: Connexions Press.

Brown, B. (2007). *I thought it was just me (but it isn't)*. New York: Penguin Random House.

Bruner, E. (1986). Ethnography as narrative. In V. Turner & E. Bruner (Eds.), *The anthropology of experience*. Chicago, IL: University of Illinois Press.

Dreikurs, R. (1967). *Psychodynamics, psychotherapy, and counseling*. Chicago, IL: Alfred Adler Institute.

Gibson, D. M., & Myers, J. E. (2000). Gender and infertility: A relational approach to counseling women. *Journal of Counseling and Development*, 78, 400–410. doi:10.1002/j.1556–6676.2000.tb01923.x.

Gottman, J. M., & Silver, N. (1999). *The seven principles for making marriage work*. New York: Three Rivers Press.

Hubble, M. A., Duncan, B. L., & Miller, S. D. (1999). *The heart & soul of change: What works in therapy*. Washington, D.C.: American Psychological Association.

Isiugo-Abanihe, U. C. (1985). Child fosterage in West Africa. *Population and Development Review*, 11, 53–73. doi:10.2307/1973378.

Jordan, J. V. (1997). Relational development through mutual empathy. In A. C. Bohart & L. S. Greenberg (Eds.), *Empathy reconsidered: New directions in psychotherapy* (pp. 343–351). Washington, D.C.: American Psychological Association.

Kaluya, R. (2014). Christian ministry and emotional health in Uganda. (Doctoral dissertation). Saint Paul School of Theology, Overland Park, KS.

Maslow, A. H. (1943). A theory of human motivation. *Psychological Review*, 50(4), 370–396. http://dx.doi.org/10.1037/h0054346.

Mugisha, J., Scholten, F., Owilla, S., Naidoo, N., Seeley, J., Chatterji, S., Kowal, P., & Boerma, T. (2013) Caregiving responsibilities and burden among older people by HIV status and other determinants in Uganda. *AIDS Care*, 25(11), 1341–1348, doi:10.1080/09540121.2013.765936.

Mujuzi, J. D. (2010). Bride wealth (price) and women's marriage – Related rights in Uganda: A historical constitutional perspective and current developments. *International Journal of Law, Policy and the Family*, 24(3). 414–430. https://doi.org/10.1093/lawfam/ebq009.

NBCC-International. (2012). Mental health facilitator program. www.nbccinternational.org/what_we_do/mhf.

Nwoye, A. (2006). A narrative approach to child and family therapy in Africa. *Contemporary Family Therapy*, 28(1) 1–23. doi:10.1007/s10591–10006–9691–9696.

Rogers, C. (1942). *Counseling and Psychotherapy: Newer concepts in practice*. Boston, MA: Houghton Mufflin Company.

Senyonyi, R. M., Ochieng, L. A., & Sells, J. (2012). The development of professional counseling in Uganda: Current status and future trends. *Journal of Counseling and Development*, 90, 500–504. doi:10.1002/j.1556–6676.2012.00062.x.

Siegel, B. (1996). African family and kinship. Anthropology Publications. Paper 3. http://scholarexchange.furman.edu/ant-publications/3.

Uganda Counseling and Support Services. (2017). Annual report. Presented at the UCSS Board Meeting April 2015. Columbia, KY.

Unicef. (2000). Domestic violence against women and girls. Innocenti Digest, 6. Retrieved from www.unicef-irc.org/publications/pdf/digest6e.pdf.

Warrington, M. (2013). Challenging the status quo: The enabling role of gender sensitive fathers, inspirational mothers, and surrogate parents in Uganda. *Educational Review*, 65, 402–415. http://dx.doi.org/10.1080/00131911.2012.689274.

White, M., & Epston, D. (1990). *Narrative means to therapeutic ends*. New York: W. W. Norton & Company.

Wolff, B., Blanc, A. K., & Gage, A. J. (2000). Who decides? Women's status and negotiation of sex in Uganda. *Culture, Health & Sexuality*, 2(3), 303–322. doi:10.1080/136910500422278.

World Health Organization. (2010). Mothering or nothing: The agony of infertility. *Bull W H O*, 88(12), 877–953. Retrieved from www.who.int/bulletin/volumes/88/12/10-011210/en/.

Additional Resources

Uganda Counseling Association. (2009). *The counsellors' code of ethics*. Kampala, Uganda: UCA.

Uganda Counseling Association: www.facebook.com/Uganda-Counselling-Association-428533443867056/.

Uganda Counseling and Support Services: www.ugandacss.org/.

Senyonyi, R. M., & Ochieng, L. A. (2012). Counseling in Uganda. In T. H. Hohenshil, N. E. Amundson, & S. G. Niles (Eds.), *Counseling around the world: An international handbook*. Alexandria, VA: American Counseling Association.

4

MARRIAGE COUNSELING WITH IRANIAN COUPLES

Neda Deylami

Overview

The aim of this chapter is to introduce localized Gottman's concepts under the theoretical framework of Gottman couple therapy that is called the Sound Relationship House Theory (SRHT) with Iranian couples. This chapter consists of three sections. The first point of focus is a brief review of information and description of divorce and the effect of its main anticipated factor – marital communication – on marital quality, and how we can improve marital communication among couples in Iran. The second section presents an outline of the Iranian culture to deepen understanding of how culture can influence on Iranian couples' interactions. Finally, this chapter ends with how a family counselor can localize Gottman's intervention for achieving a more effective couple intervention.

Main Anticipated Factors of Divorce

In general, humankind tends to gain well-being through developing and maintaining romantic and close relationships and forming families through marriage. Marriage is the most fundamental relationship in a family institution especially among Muslim population in which provide majority of emotional, psychological, and financial well-being with specific advantages, for instance, longevity, deeper happiness, a higher level of physical and emotional as well as sexual satisfaction (Askari, 2010), greater career satisfaction and more financial earnings (Kreager, Felson, Warner, & Wenger, 2013), lower rates of domestic abuse experiences (Cornelius, Shorey, & Beebe, 2010) and more wealth. Nevertheless, low marital quality inhibits the advantages of marriage and often leads to divorce.

Since the 1960s, there has been a sudden and sharp decline in marriage rates and the dramatically increased rate of divorce throughout the world has provided the severe psychological and financial costs for both families and societies (Bodenmann, Pihet, Shantinath, Cina, & Widmer, 2006). Divorce and dissolution as well as emotional disengagement have provided a majority of social, psychological, financial, and legal problems for Iranian and non-Iranian couples and society as well. The social illness of divorce has high prevalence in Muslim countries (Dommaraju & Jones, 2011). Although Islam considers divorce as the necessary evil, and divorce is permissible, it is still very much discouraged, unless it has become a threat to the married couple. Islam considers marriage is a better choice than divorce and remaining single.

The divorce rate in Malaysia as a Muslim country that is aiming towards a developed nation by the year 2020 has reached 22% among married couples from 18 to 50 years old (Hassan, 2015). Added to that, divorce in the Kingdom of Saudi Arabia happens at the rate of 127 cases per day, or about five cases every hour. It is worth noting that 60% of divorce cases occur in the first year of marriage. This has been revealed in a report by the General Authority of Statistics of Kingdom of Saudi Arabia (2015). It is striking that Indonesian couples with their Muslim marriages get divorced, on average, more than 1,000 cases per day (Nurlaelawati, 2013). The roots of these changes are in the demographic transition arising out of the social and economic developments of the last century.

Similarly, the divorce rate in Iran is substantial. Iran has the highest growth rate of divorce among Islamic countries in the Middle East and North Africa region (Aghajanian & Thompson, 2013). The National Organization for Civil Registration in Iran (2015) has reported that divorce occurs 18 times per hour. Iranians are witnessing the steadily increasing trend of the divorce rate. The recorded divorces in Iran were 155,369 cases in 2014, while marriage rates have declined in the last three and half years, down by 1.9% in 2012; 5.1% in 2013; 6.7% in 2014; and 7.2% in the first half of 2015 (Iran's Ministry of Interior, 2015).

The skyrocketing divorce rate in Iran in Iranian families in recent decades may be attributed to social changes, historical transitions, and a range of socio-economic, cultural, and religious factors such as modernization, the 1979 Islamic revolution, and a destructive eight-year war between Iran and Iraq (Farmam & Pakgohar, 2011; Aghajanian & Thompson, 2013). It has been noted that differences in our previous traditional histories and modern socio-political movements and levels of industrial-economic development create the conditions for Iranian women to experience gender oppression. Based on these factors and a report from the National Organization for Civil Registration in Iran (Iran's Ministry of Interior, 2015), Iranian families have faced social changes, including an increase of the average marriage age. From 2005 to 2014, the percentage of unmarried men older than 35 rose from 6.7% to 10.2%. In the same period, the percentage of unmarried women over 30 increased from 6.3% to 13.8%. The accustomed marriage age at the said year ranged from 20 to 34 for men and 15 to 29 for women.

Researchers emphasize that separation and divorce have strong and significant negative consequences for the mental and physical health of both spouses, not just for the one who requested to get divorce. These negative effects include an increased risk for psychopathology, an increased number of automobile accidents, suicide, and homicide as well as violence. It appears that an improvement in marital quality and prevention of separation and divorce is a concern of every society.

A relationship in marriage does not occur in a vacuum but depends on the interaction between couples' interpersonal skills such as marital communication, intrapersonal characteristics, personal experiences, family of-origin background and a set of socio-economic-cultural factors (Halford, Markman, Kling, & Stanley, 2003; Sanders, 2010). Couples can learn how they are able to change and enhance these factors. Navarra (2011) suggests that the main predictor cause of the rise in divorce rates and marital dissolutions is the lack of dyadic competencies, such as communication skills, conflict management, problem-solving capacities, and emotional engagement in both partners. To prevent dissolution and divorce; attendance in education programs, counseling, or family therapy for achieving above-mentioned skills is vital.

Among all, marital communication is considered as a central component and a major predictor of marital quality. The abilities to communicate effectively and manage conflict are critical to increasing marital satisfaction which is related to general happiness and pleasure (Edalati & Redzuan, 2010). The accumulated data (Askari, 2010; Blanchard, Hawkins, Baldwin, & Fawcett, 2009; Gottman, 2014; Gottman & Swanson, 2002; J. M. Gottman & Gottman, 2011; Kalantarkousheh, Hassan, Kadir, & Talib, 2011) illustrate that the quality of reciprocal communication between husbands and wives was highly predictive of marital distress or divorce. A long-lasting marriage will be achieved if couples attend family education training programs, learn marital communication skills and do their best accordingly to improve their own intrapersonal characteristics and other relevant interpersonal skills (Sanders, 2010).

Communication problems are one of the sources of highest conflict for couples (Gottman, 2014), making it the most commonly reported problem by couples seeking professional help to rebuild their marital life (Gurman, Lebow, & Snyder, 2015). Obviously, insufficient marital knowledge and low quality of dyadic interaction between couples can deconstruct the marital relationships and lead to dissolution and divorce. Family researchers (Blanchard et al., 2009; Askari, Noah, Hassan, & Baba, 2012) indicated the necessity of marital communication skills training for prevention of marital problems and divorce. On the other hand, recent developments in family counseling have heightened the necessity of couples' training and family education programs instead of family therapy (Sillars, Canary, & Vangelisti, 2013; Woszidlo & Segrin, 2013).

Similar to non-Iranian couples, Iranian couples must learn how to create and maintain marital satisfaction by marital communication skills, which can be developed either by attending counseling sessions or couples' training programs. Simultaneously, many studies, to prevent a dramatic increase of divorce in Iran, studied the effectiveness of family interventions on marital communication because of the significant deficiencies in previous researches on family therapy (Deylami, Khalatbari, & Hashemian, 2007; Hosseinkhanzadeh, & Yeganeh, 2013; Rakhshani, Niknami, & Ansari Moghadam, 2005). Consequently, couples with relevant marital knowledge can regulate affection, manage conflicts, and achieve health and happiness more than couples who are in discordant marriages and avoid learning these skills (Ebrahimi & Kimiaei, 2014; Proulx, Helms, & Buehler, 2007).

The family knowledge and couples' skills, like declaration of intimacy and admiration, management of conflict and problem solving can help Iranian couples improve and maintain their marital quality and prevent of other marital maladjustment such as domestic violence or infidelity (Madahi, Samadzadeh, & Javidi, 2013). Although maintenance of marital quality is not an easy task, psychological research shows that researched-based marital education programs can help couples maintain their marital quality to be effective and making unhappy marriages more satisfying. Evidence from a study of Iranian couples who participated in preventive or psycho-educational training programs suggests that training can have an effect on improvement of marital satisfaction and, thus, decrease divorce rates (Askari, 2010; Kalantarkousheh et al., 2011). However, training by any intervention without considering cultural, local, and social norms and values might be problematic for audiences, because they may learn skills and principles that conflict with their values. Hence, the most important responsibility of any Iranian family counselor is to find an effective couple therapy with low relapse rate and integrated approach to couple therapy and also low clash rate with Iranian-Islamic culture.

The Gottman's psycho-educational intervention that is under the theory of the Sound Relationship House Theory (SRHT) might be a good selection for maintenance of marital quality and strengthening marriages for couples (Gottman, 2014). It is an effective intervention for couples. SRHT is an evidence-based treatment that can train couples to achieve all relevant marital skills with a low relapse rate of less than 20%. This relapse rate might be very significant for family counselors because Gottman shows a 60% relapse rate for couples who refer to very high qualified family counselors, and they divorce as soon as finishing the intervention (J.M. Gottman & Gottman, 2010). The low relapse rate in Gottman therapy (just only 20%) deals with couple conflict and resolution and even beyond of conflict, emphasizing the couple's intimacy and improving their loves and friendship as well as creating the shared meaning system (Gottman, 2011).

It is expected by this intervention that couples learn how to be more validating and non-judgmental of each other, to enhance their own emotions positively and regulate their emotional expressions, and manage their conflicted issues (Henderson, Robey, Dunham, & Dermer, 2013). Furthermore, couples, by Gottman's psycho-educational intervention, learn how they can express their empathy and understanding of each other and show the art and science of love (Gurman, Lebow, & Snyder, 2015). They will be able to strengthen the emotional engagement – attachment – in their relationship. This intervention is a research-based approach that is designed in an educational, skill training model. However, as long as conducting Gottman therapy for achieving the more long-lasting results, the family counselors must recognize cultural considerations and the social values systems of clients. Therefore, any attitude towards families should benefit from the new generation's attitude towards the concept of family as well as the society values (Edalati & Redzuan, 2010).

Iranian Culture and Iranian Couples

Iran is a Middle Eastern country, an Islamic republic on the Persian Gulf with historical sites dating back to the Persian Empire. It shares Islam as a religion with other countries in the region. The nation is one of the largest and most influential countries in the Middle East with multi-ethnics and multi-cultures that had always followed monotheism. Regarding to statistical Center of Iran (2015), over 99% of Iranians are Muslim, and a very limited number of Jews and Armenians. Islam is practiced by the majority of Iranians and governs their personal, political, economic, and legal lives. The most important ethnic groups are the Persians, Turks, Baluchi, Arabs, and Kurds. The majority of Iranian people are Shi'ite Moslems, which is significantly different from the Sunni sect that is followed by most of the Arab countries of the Middle East. The strong, rich, and ancient civilization in Iran began in the pre-Islamic era and inherited the Persian culture and language in which belong to 7,000 years ago (Daniel, 2012).

Historically, Iranians have been monotheists, believing in the oneness of God, and followed the pre-Islamic Zoroastrian religion; as a result, Iranian cultural values and Islamic values are typically harmonious. Iran emerged as a significant regional power after conversion to Islam and made many great contributions to literature, philosophy, and science. However, Iran transformed into the 20th century with an underdeveloped economy and weak central government.

Added to traditional-religious approach, since 100 years ago, some national and international factors such as establishing the Ministry of Education (1910), the post-World War II period (1955–1979), the rapid economic growth and modernization due to oil exports, and social reforms (1936), influenced Iranian family institution and the status of women. These modernizing and Westernizing factors changed the social status of women and increased their participation in social and economic domains outside the household. These changes granted the right to vote and increased the political participation for women, placing them in high positions within the government bureaucracy (Aghajanian, 2001). Pursuant to these social changes, the family laws were improved, enhancing women's situations within marriage and family.

The Islamic revolution of 1979 was a turning point in the social and economic history of Iran. It is considered as one of the most important events to take place in the Middle East within the past 60 years. Iran has experienced the dramatic and meaningful social, economic, and political transformations that have led to renewed attention to the ways in which social interaction and cultural tradition have evolved. Iran is currently experiencing long-term processes of cumulative social changes across society that have developed various kinds of reactions and adjustments (Aghajanian, 2001). It is a transitional period with many social values having been transformed.

Another important change in Iranian family structure is based on the higher chance for women to earn incomes and acquire property. Recently, Iranian women have become a larger percentage of the formal labor force than in the past, more often attaining post-graduation education, are more active in society, and have increased their share of ownership of property and business (Aghajanian, 2001). As a result, the educational achievement and earning money among women have markedly influenced the increasing age of marriage in recent years (Aghajanian & Thompson, 2013). As women become more aware of their right and try to employ it, this would lead to higher number of divorces for women, where they are in abusive marriage relationships (Edalati & Redzuan, 2010; Aghajanian & Thompson, 2013).

The changing of family structure in terms of its size and direction is another aspect of transformation in Iran. Previously, about one-third of Iranian family size was an extended family, while nowadays more than 85% live in nuclear families combined of parents and children only or even sometimes just only one parent with one child. Also, the family direction has been changed; some families follow modernity and Western culture, while the others are influenced and very restricted to obey of traditional and religious directions. The family structure has been influenced from both legal and social changes (Edalati & Redzuan, 2010).

In comparing traditional Iranian family structures with modern families, significant issues have emerged. Women have been protected and taken care of by men. It has been inappropriate to ask questions about an Iranian's wife or other female relatives. Their loyalty to the family is paramount. The relationship between the husband and wife relationship has been largely based on differing gender roles. The history of Iran is known as masculine-dominant and masculine-oriented (Father/husband-oriented) history (Gokturk & Arslan, 2010).

Iranian families have been dominated by fathers. For instance, children would have the father's surname, and in the traditional family the son would typically continue in his father's line of work. Fathers make decisions for future marriages of the family members (Edalati & Redzuan, 2010). The father works to support the family, and if he is unable to find a job, there is enormous stress exerted on the marriage. The man may seem like a failure, and will express his inner emotions through anger. Islamic values and teachings have shaped Iranian society for many centuries, and continue to support the patriarchal family framework.

Recent developments in Iranian family structure led to renewed interest and prime concern among Iranian women in the new generation. Although women have typically contributed to the economic activity of the family via domestically generated income within the household, many desire to work on a parity with men outside of the home (Aghajanian & Thompson, 2013). Many women of this new generation would like to follow modernity, so Iranian women nowadays are faced with occupational opportunities. They have high level of education in modern society and would like to participate in outside social activities and earn incomes. This may reveal the reason why the marriage age has increased (Sadeghi & Kalhor, 2007).

This modern trend is often in conflict with their fathers' and husbands' traditional point of view. Traditionally, they were not enthusiastic about women working outside of the house. The traditional family structure has always supported the idea of domestic responsibilities as a woman's primary role for "a good woman" and the role of men in the dominant economic position of "breadwinner" for "a responsible man" (Khosravi et al., 2007).

This traditional family context has been consistent with the teachings of Islam, as much as the Iranian socio-cultural system and Islamic penal codes encourage men to be responsible in family life: controlling property, the guardianship of children legally, and restricting their wives' public activities are men's rights (Moghissi, 2016). Women are forced to obey their husbands. It is emphasized that women must be good wives and raise generations of good Moslems. Yet Islam does not prohibit non-household roles for women. A married woman may be gainfully employed; however, if her husband doesn't permit her, or the nature of her occupation is not compatible with her family's interest or dignity, the husband may prevent his wife from participating in such an occupation. While the job situation and salary can be a guarantee source for women in their old age crisis, this saving is important for them because regarding to the Islamic inheritance law, men inherit two times more than women (Hoodfar & Assadpour, 2000). Actually, women have limited access to divorce and fewer inheritance rights than men. Patriarchy and other forms of male dominance are emphasized by this kind of law and even modern family law. Regarding these laws, men's power over women will be increased maximally. As a result, women's ability to make decisions and independent action will limited and decrease.

It is generally considered these modern social changes currently alter gender roles, compared to previous generations. Acceptance of dependency and a husband-oriented affiliation have changed for wives; many women believe they can be independent and do not need their husbands. The gender role of "financial supporter" and "male breadwinner" for husbands is changed due to the change the women's social status and increasing the chance of earn money for wives. Regarding the modern point of view among women, the primary roles of motherhood and wife have changed for many couples, which may place couples at greater risk of marital dissolution and divorce, according to reports from Iranian family courts (Khosravi et al., 2007).

In general, therefore, it seems that Iranian family structure and the status of women and men in the family have been influenced by both legal changes and social changes. Taken together, these changes increased the marriage age from 14 to 15–29 years of age for females and 16 to 20–34 years of age for males. According to The National Organization for Civil Registration in Iran (2013), the common age of marriage is 20 to 34 years for men and 15 to 29 years for women. In the 2013, the rate of marriage for males who were passing the common age of marriage was 9.4%, while this rate increased to 10.4% in 2014. Moreover, in 2013, the frequency of females who passed common age increased from 12.5% in 2013 to 14.5% in 2014. Additionally, on the other hand the divorce rate has been increased.

Recently, Iranian family counselors and sociologists have drawn the transitional period influence on the divorce issue. Currently, after many changes, those couples who have mutually agreed to divorce are allowed to go to an office of notary public, called the Mahzar, and register their divorce in front of two witnesses. To protect women against coercive consent to divorce, the law was recently modified to give women the special chance to submit their petition to court if they disagreed with the divorce. It is important to note that the availability of modern technology and virtual-cybernetic communications, as well as the expansion of mass media, has speeded up the diffusion of non-Iranian culture among younger generations (Aghajanian & Thompson, 2013).

Iranian Localization of Gottman's Psycho-Educational Intervention

In recent years, couples typically request marital counseling or attend a family education program during significant developmental milestones (birth, sickness, death, children's entry into school or graduation, onset of puberty, etc.) and during significant life changes (retirement, employment transition, relocation, migration, etc.) for marital support. Gottman's psycho-education intervention has been shown to be one of the most effective interventions for solution of family problems (Gottman & Silver, 2012; Gottman, 2016). Gottman introduces three important skills in his intervention that couples need to learn for having constructive communication and avoiding destructive ones for successful marital quality: 1) how to prevent conflict whenever possible; 2) how to reach an agreement and ensure positive dialogue during an unavoidable conflict; and 3) how to recover when partners become distanced from each other (J. M. Gottman & Gottman, 2011).

Gottman suggests for prevention of divorce, and any marital problems, both spouses have to learn marital skills by attending either counseling-therapeutic sessions or training sessions (Gottman, 2016); however, far too little attention has been paid to localization of Gottman's psycho-educational intervention for improving of marital communication in Iran. Iranian couples are rarely inclined towards couple therapy. Indeed, among Iranians, training is more preferable as compared to family therapy or counseling. "Training" is a preferable alternative for them. However, Iranian spouses still have low attendance in family training programs specially, with each other. They usually want to attend training sessions alone without their spouses. It has to be noted that both individual couples and cultural differences must be considered, with some of Gottman's concepts needing to be culturally localized.

Case Example

Sara was referred to a counseling center as a result of maladjustment. She is suffering from a troubled marriage and her decision in the first session was to seek a divorce. She is 28 years old and has already achieved her master's degree in civil engineering. She is a first child and her parents are lecturers in university and her two siblings are graduated with master's degrees. Sara's parents are validating and, Sara believes, wish to negotiate and demand on family issues for future solving of problems. Sara has been married for 2 years to Ahmad who is dentist and 38 years of age. Both have no children. Ahmad's father works at a traditional market in Shiraz, while her mother is house-maker and responsible for Ahmad's other four siblings. Ahmad's family of-origin is very restricted about traditional norms and they don't allow the family women to work and continue their study. His family type is a conflict avoider with very rigid and clear boundaries. No fight, no demand, just follow the role and hierarchy. Since the early months of Sara's marriage, she has faced many marital conflicts without any successful attempts to solve them. Ahmad is used to contempt and ridicule his wife and neglect her in front of his family. Ahmad is very dependent on his family and unable to make decisions independently even in the very private marital issues such as permission for Sara's job. Although Sara has found a full-time job as an assistant in a corporate car factory, her husband has not allowed her to work. Sara is emotionally abused by her husband with his humiliating criticism and mocking manners. However, after every bad conflict her husband feels very regretful, promising this is the last time and asks for another chance. Sara believes in his love and passion but she cannot tolerate his disrespectful behavior. Sara has been physically abused by her husband with slaps on her face, push and intimidation in sex. However she has avoided talking about these matters with anyone.

Sara has requested divorce twice already and has referred to the family court; however, in accordance with Iranian-Islamic Civil Code Article 1132: A man can refer to the conditions provided by the law courts for divorce. In general, women could not divorce. Unless there are defects in the case of a man with flaws like a mad man and impotency provided that even once the marriage is not done or amputation of the penis to the extent that is not able to have sexual relations. Regarding Sara's lack of legal proof, the judge didn't accept her request for divorce. The judge can only accept her complaints about domestic violence – only physical abuse not sexual or emotional – with the condition of her providing enough legal evidence from neighbors and any relatives. Finally, he advised Sara it is better to come back to family and continue her marital life because her husband is not guilty of any "social accepted bad traits," such as addiction, infidelity, sodomy, and depravity or any antisocial behavior. Additionally, the judge recommended her to ask the court to terminate the contract of employment, not to file for divorce. Sara faced a paradox: she was unable to show convincing evidence and worried about her family's honor, and on the other hand she loved her husband and hoped to construct their marital life, and deeply wanted to finish this dissolution and prevent of divorce in the future.

Therefore, she refers to a family counseling center, but alone. I try to help her with asking myself: under what circumstances, the intimate partner violence is justifiable between two spouses? And basically, my answer is that any types of domestic violence are unacceptable in an intimate relationship. While, in reality, I consulted a person who attends the counseling session, loves her husband and does not accept or tolerate the violence, on the other side, I'm faced with an abusive person who is refusing to attend a counseling session especially with a female counselor and labels his aggressive behaviors as male chauvinism and loves his wife. For helping this couple and due to the potential ethical, moral, cultural, and legal conditions, I am unable to consider directly this case as an intimate partner violence, hence, I have to utilize another brilliant and indirect concept and strategy like Gottman theory as an effective psycho-educational intervention to assist her for prevention of dissolution and encourage her husband to attend the therapeutic / psycho-educational intervention …

Consultation with Sara

Sara expressed her chief complaints, and I realized that my client's problem is a kind of maladjusted marital interaction. There is a risk when individual counseling is exclusively employed to address a relationship complaint and problematic interaction patterns.

The effective counseling rule: The counselor and Gottman therapist should consider the reciprocal interaction between spouses and not emphasize individual counseling.

The Gottman's concept: Gottman focuses on "changing interaction patterns" and how couples think about their relationship, and how they feel about feelings. Therefore both spouses attending is necessary to get the best results. The couple are a good example of a dyad. Everything which occurred in the marital family due to the wife's attitude can affect her own characteristics as well as her husband's characteristics. Additionally, the husband's attitude will be affected by his own characteristics as well as by his wife's characteristics. This reciprocal interaction and non-independence is significant when there is an effect of relationships on individuals' behaviors, perceptions, feelings, and attitudes. Therefore, if it is ignored by a counselor, the potential ability for "change" will be lost and will limit the results for couple-level relationships (Ackerman, Donnellan, & Kashy, 2011; Cook & Kenny, 2005).

Iranian localized concept: To localize the concept of "changing interaction patterns," some thoughtful strategies are needed. When the spouses enter into the relationship with one another, they try to form a unique meta-emotion combination, while in the ailing relationship, meta-emotion mismatches have often disrupted their interaction. It is most probably impossible if the counselor wants to help couples when just only one of them is attending the therapeutic session because you as a counselor just encounter with one meat-emotion system and you have no chance to mediate it and change interaction patterns.

Basically, to have both spouses in the family counseling sessions is a significant challenge for many Iranian family counselors (Honarian, Younesi, Shafiabadi, & Nafissi, 2010; Fereydoni, Tabrizi, & Nejad, 2009). The Iranian husband is usually unwilling to attend a counseling center and even in the family education programs which are very common in education system (such as schools in all levels both public and private ones, others educational centers in municipalities, and universities). The husband often balks counselor recommendations by providing many excuses. Sometimes he believes there is no need to attend counseling sessions because the marital problems do not belong to him, or are totally those are his wife. Or he thinks attending the counseling session is wasting time and money without any real and long-lasting effects.

The family counselor must be aware that although traditionally the husband believes he is responsible for the family, he reluctantly accepts the blame for his responsibility for mistakes and problems. Hence, no need to stimulate the guilty and worthless feelings. Most probably he will accept your invitation to attend, and then you as a creative counselor have to pay very careful attention to the quality of the therapeutic alliance. You have been able to form so far with each of them. You must be convinced that there is an atmosphere of caring and respect, even love (humanitarian not sexual), that you develop for both spouses. Only in a caring atmosphere can the couple safety feel to dive into the deep understanding of their marital issues, to be brave for acceptance of change and attempt to solve their problems.

Issue: Sara faces three important conflict topics including finance (conflict over money), "in-low" issues, and intimacy (complaining about passion, admiration, sex, and physical/emotional abusing).

My challenge: Sarah experiences physical violence in the relationship. All my therapeutic strategies have to be arranged around intimate partner violence issue.

The effective counseling rule: Any question or decision regarding a client's marital status belongs to the client – not the counselor. To have more accurate information and future therapeutic steps, the interview and assessment with both spouses is essential (Weeks & Fife, 2014).

Iranian localized concept: Definitely, the Iranian family counselor as others must consider saying or doing everything with the client with a therapeutic intent. Nothing should be random or incidental when interacting with the client, especially when the clients are a couple. The counselors need to have information and deepen understanding of underlying dynamics of the conflicts; sometimes Iranian counselors spend a lot of time and many therapeutic sessions to obtain the information. Basically, Iranian counselors must know regarding to Gottman (2010) without formal assessment of the relationship and accurate evaluation of client's problem before beginning treatment will lead to psychotherapy errors. On the other hand, Iranian clients have a lack of patients to attend many sessions, because of financial issues, job responsibilities, and family budget. Consequently, utilizing the triple steps of interview and evaluation by Gottman's scales instead of immediate treatment with spending many sessions is appropriate for Iranian culture. It can provide more accurate information for counselors and will be very interesting for Iranian clients because it saves time and money for them. A careful assessment by Gottman's scales in the beginning of treatment can help Iranian counselors to give the couple feedback about their marital relationship, building the couple's expectations, formulate the therapeutic objectives, and discuss where to start and how the intervention will be work (Gottman, 2011). The time will be very spent and the counselor and Gottman therapist will be building a deep therapeutic alliance. Hence, assessment can modify the counselor's orientation and perception about the client's issues and prevent the future diagnostics mistakes.

Issue: Sara and her husband disagree with their partner's different attitudes about one of the most important marital issues is called "power control." They blame each other and agitate.

My challenge: Totally, moving beyond blame and defensiveness is essential to the creation of a therapeutic environment in which both spouses equally can safely experiment with new paths of power control. However, Ahmad and Sara, like the majority of Iranian couples, disagree with each other in this issue and every one would like to be winner in the "power struggle" and cannot be patient to change.

Iranian localized concept: Many Iranian men are against the power-sharing concept. These traditional and religious persons believe men must be managers and that supervision is men's right, emphasized by the Quran (Al-Nisa, verse 34), while they have a misunderstanding of the Quran's approach about the men's fair power. Islam is the source of civil law in our country. Family is considered as a contiguous system that has to have only one leader and this leadership is granted to men. Let it be noted that in Iran, issues related to men's authority and his right of family management are both lawful and legitimate. According to the Civil Code of the Islamic Republic of Iran, in Article 1105, after contracting marriage, being the head of the family is the characteristic and responsibility of the husband. But some men behave with authoritarian management because of the lack of understanding of the concept of men management due to the dominant culture.

The family counselor must enlighten each couple specially the husband, even if the men are supposed to be head of the family, in the religious approach; this position does not allow him to be lordly. It asks him not only to be a leader but a servant as well. He must cooperate with the other members in that system. Therefore, as an effective manager, he should consult with his wife and other family members and use their advice. There is no doubt, without any appropriate abilities nobody can manage and direct a system.

Iranian localized concept: Regarding the Islamic approach and management sciences, irregularities and chaos are the basic problems in an organization with two leaders and heads without clear boundaries and without appropriate limitations. These issues are not very strange and new to the majority of men who are already following traditional and religious values. No doubt they believe the responsibility, leadership, and management of the family should be left to the man, and he must be the head of the family because of his physical and psychological structure. Here a misunderstanding exists, and men often get their benefits with hierarchy and autarchy. They emphasize that men lead women because of the excellence that God has for some, more than others, and because they spend their property on women's alimony (Mir-Hosseini, 2006).

On the other side, women's greater involvement in higher education and labor community has brought the attitude variation towards traditional marital roles, family values, and difficulties in compromising roles within their marital life (Sadeghi & Kalhor, 2007).

My challenge: My determined question is whether the partner's intimate violence in this case is regarding to the influence and interference of husband's family of-origin structure or even his attachment style, or other intrapersonal factors, or whether it is based on the ineffective relationship patterns like lack of acceptance of their influence? Do I have to focus on changing the violated symptoms or improving their marital interaction with increasing their positivity and deescalate their negativity?

The effective counseling rule: The family counselor should consider a protocol for distinguishing "solvable problems" from some other marital problems, which those are perpetual and not easy to solve. The counselor must realize that in classifying the topics of discussions of major areas of continuing disagreement, 69% of the time couples are talking about a perpetual problem (Gottman, 2010) that they had had in their relationship for many years, such as their family of-origin issues. Therefore, find the solvable problems, concentrate on perpetual issues.

Iranian localized concept: This concept is approved by well-educated, professional Iranian women. They can accept the influence of their husbands and turn toward their bids, without any reservations or negativity. The counselor and Gottman therapist must teach the couple the importance of this concept. It is very important for both spouses to follow, but some Iranian husbands sometimes cannot grasp the meaning of influence to prevent dissolution. This element as easily affects wives because of some hidden social forces.

The family counselor must enlighten each couple, especially the husband; this concept does not mean compliance. This is avoidance of prejudice and is the component of "give and take," of reasonableness, and of compromise. Hence, compromise in finding a common ground for "yes" has its roots in the very beginning of a problem's discussion and prevention of escalating of negative emotion and violent behavior.

Overall, other concepts in Gottman's intervention, like "Friendship, Admiration, De-escalation and Prevention of four horsemen ("Criticism, Defensiveness, Contempt, and Stonewalling") are the main concepts in family life that are strictly reinforced by Islamic and Iranian cultural approaches. It is written in the Quran (Rome, verse 21) that the woman is a significant source of relief, peace in mind, and calmness for men. Since the couple need gravity and heart transplants, the verse says: "and he created between you 'Rahma' and 'Mavada'": that means love and mercy. These elements are accepted for women and men based on their cultural and religious values. Traditionally, Iranians have learned to respect elder people as well as authorized people like the husband in family; to follow and obey the hierarchy is historically reinforced in Iran.

A concept of "Repair Attempts" is the last concept that, compared to the Islamic-Iranian culture, is very important in Gottman's method, not only for improving the friendship between couples but also improving the duration of conflict and affects after the conflict. Both Islam and Iranian culture strongly advise couples to attempt to repair their relationship with each other and to individually control negativity.

Handling aggression and negative feelings and self-smoothing are very recognized behaviors among couple relationships that reach the highest levels of friendship. This concept is emphasized in the Quran: "And of his signs is that you have created spouses of your own selves (not of angels and not of goblins and others), to be peaceful with them, and between you (woman and human beings), friendship and love inwardly, there are signs (in God's wisdom and power and wisdom) for the people who are thinking" (Rome, verse: 21).

Summary

This chapter was only one step to localize a very significant couple therapy (Gottman therapy has only 20% relapse rate) for counseling society of Iran. It might be useful for either Iranian counselors or non-Iranian counselors with counseling of Iranian clients. Furthermore, it might motivate non-Iranian counselors to localize this great approach (Gottman's psycho-educational intervention) with their own culture to address this question how traditional effects can influence the family functioning and the process of therapeutic attempts.

References

Ackerman, R. A., Donnellan, M. B., & Kashy, D. A. (2011). Working with dyadic data in studies of emerging adulthood: Specific recommendations, general advice, and practical tips. In F. D. Fincham & M. Cui (Eds.), *Romantic relationships in emerging adulthood* (pp. 67–97). New York: Cambridge University Press.

Aghajanian, A. (2001). Family and family change in Iran. (Doctoral dissertation). Retrieved from www.faculty.uncfsu.edu (28301).

Aghajanian, A., & Thompson, V. (2013). Recent divorce trend in Iran. *Journal of Divorce & Remarriage, 54*(2), 112–125. doi:10.1080/10502556.2012.752687.

Arcuri. (2013). Dyadic perfectionism, communication patterns and relationship quality in couples. (Doctoral dissertation). Retrieved from Electronic Theses and Dissertations (4940). http://scholar.uwindsor.ca/etd/4940.

Arroyo, A., & Segrin, C. (2011). The relationship between self-and other-perceptions of communication competence and friendship quality. *Communication Studies*, 62(5), 547–562. doi:10.1080/10510974.2011.580037.

Askari, M. (2010). Effects of communication and conflict resolution skills training on marital satisfaction and mental health among Iranian couples. (Unpublished doctoral dissertation). UPM, Malaysia.

Askari, M., Noah, S., Hassan, S., & Baba, M. (2012). Comparison the effects of communication and conflict resolution skills training on marital satisfaction. *International Journal of Psychological Studies*, 4(1), 182.

Blanchard, V. L., Hawkins, A. J., Baldwin, S. A., & Fawcett, E. B. (2009). Investigating the effects of marriage and relationship education on couples' communication skills: A meta-analytic study. *Journal of Family Psychology*, 23(2), 203. Retrieved from doi:10.1037/a0015211.

Bodenmann, G., Pihet, S., Shantinath, S. D., Cina, A., & Widmer, K. (2006). Improving dyadic coping in couples with a stress-oriented approach: A 2-year longitudinal study. *Behavior Modification*, 30(5), 571–597.

Cook, W. L., & Kenny, D. A. (2005). The actor–partner interdependence model: A model of bidirectional effects in developmental studies. *International Journal of Behavioral Development*, 29(2), 101–109. doi:10.1080/01650250444000405.

Cornelius, T. L., Shorey, R. C., & Beebe, S. M. (2010). Self-reported communication variables and dating violence: Using Gottman's marital communication conceptualization. *Journal of Family Violence*, 25(4), 439–448.

Daniel, E. L. (2012). The history of Iran, ABC-CLIO. Retrieved from www.books.google.com.

Deylami, N., Khalatbari, J., & Hashemian, K. (2007). Relationship between attachment style and family structure with domestic violence: Effect of marital life training on domestic violence among Iranian couple in Tehran University dormitories (Unpublished master's thesis). Science and Research Azad University, Tehran, Iran.

Dommaraju, P. & Jones, G. (2011). Divorce trends in Asia. *Asian Journal of Social Science*, 39 (6), 725–750.

Ebrahimi, E., & Kimiaei, A. (2014). The study of the relationship among marital satisfaction, attachment styles, and communication patterns in divorcing couples. *Journal of Divorce & Remarriage*, 55(6), 451–463. doi:10.1093/jpepsy/jss063.

Edalati, A., & Redzuan, M. R. (2010). Perception of women towards family values and their marital satisfaction. *Journal of American Science*, 6(4): 132–137.

Farmam, F. A., & Pakgohar, M. (2011). Effect of pre-marriage counselling on marital satisfaction of Iranian newlywed couples: A randomized controlled trial. *Sexuality & Culture*, 15(2), 141–152.

Fereydoni, K. J., Tabrizi, M., & Nejad, S. N. (2009). The impact "self regulation brief couple therapy" increases couple's satisfaction in the clients of Babolsar Farhangian Clinic. *Journal of Family Research*, 4(3), 213–229.

Gokturk, S., & Arslan, H. (2010). The effects of cultural values on the quality of mentoring relationship. *International Journal of Educational Researchers*, 1(3), 31–42.

Gottman, J. M. (2014). *Principia amoris: The new science of love*: New York: Routledge.

Gottman, J. M. (2016). *Men in marriages and families*. New York: Psychology Press.

Gottman, J. M., & Gottman, J. S. (2010). *Bridging the couple chasm*. Plano, TX: Southern Methodist University Department of Dispute Resolution and Counseling.

Gottman, J. M., & Gottman, J. S. (2011). *Bridging the couple therapy; Gottman couples therapy: A research-based approach*. Seattle, WA: Gottman Institute.

Gottman, J., & Silver, N. (2012). *What Makes Love Last?: How to build trust and avoid betrayal*. New York: Simon & Schuster.

Gottman, J. M., & Swanson, C. (2002). A general systems theory of marriage: Nonlinear difference equation modeling of marital interaction. *Personality and Social Psychology Review*, 6(4), 326–340.

Gurman, A. S., Lebow, J. L., & Snyder, D. K. (2015). *Clinical handbook of couple therapy*. New York: The Guilford Press.

Halford, W. K., Markman, H. J., Kling, G. H., & Stanley, S. M. (2003). Best practice in couple relationship education. *Journal of Marital and Family Therapy*, 29(3), 385–406. Retrieved from http://search.proquest.com.

Hassan, S. A. (2015). Islamic transcendental wellbeing model for Malaysian Muslim women: Implication on counselling. *Asian Social Science*, 11(21). doi:10.5539/ass.v11n21p331.

Henderson, A., Robey, P., Dunham, S., & Dermer, S. (2013). Change, choice, and home: An integration of the work of Glasser and Gottman. *International Journal of Choice Theory and Reality Therapy*, 32(2), 36.

Honarian, M., Younesi, J., Shafiabadi, A., & Nafissi, G. (2010). "The impact of couple therapy based on attachment" in deterministic thinking and marital satisfaction among couples. *International Journal of Psychology and Counselling*, 2, 91–99.

Hoodfar, H., & Assadpour, S. (2000). The politics of population policy in the Islamic Republic of Iran. *Studies in Family Planning* 31(1), 19–34.

Hosseinkhanzadeh, A. A., & Yeganeh, T. (2013). The effects of life skills training on marital satisfaction. *Procedia-Social and Behavioral Sciences*, 84, 769–772.

Iran's Minstry of Interior, National Organization of Civil Registration (NOCR). (2015). Vital statistics events. Retrieved from www.sciencedirect.com.

Kalantarkousheh, S. M., Hassan, A. S., Kadir, R. A., & Talib, M. A. (2011). Efficiency of the existential time training on the marital satisfaction among the Iranian women. *Procedia Social and Behavioral Sciences*. Retrieved from http://works.bepress.com/siti_hassan/21/.

Khosravi, A., Taylor, R., Naghavi, M., & Lopez, A. D. (2007). Mortality in the Islamic Republic of Iran, 1964–2004. *Bulletin of the World Health Organization,* 85(8), 607–614. doi:10.1590/S0042–96862007000800013.

Kingdom of Saudi Arabia. (2015). The general authority of statistics. Vital Statistics Events. Retrieved from http://www.stats.gov.sa/en.

Kreager, D. A., Felson, R. B., Warner, C., & Wenger, M. R. (2013). Women's education, marital violence, and divorce: A social exchange perspective. *Journal of Marriage and Family*, 75(3), 565–581.

Madahi, M. E., Samadzadeh, M., & Javidi, N. (2013). The communication patterns & satisfaction in married students. *Procedia-Social and Behavioral Sciences*, 84, 1190–1193. doi:10.1016/j.sbspro.2013.06.725.

Mir-Hosseini, Z. (2006). Muslim women's quest for equality: Between Islamic law and feminism. *Critical Inquiry*, 32(4), 629–645.

Moghissi, H. (1996). *Populism and feminism in Iran: Women's struggle in a male-defined revolutionary movement*. Basingstoke: Palgrave Macmillan.
Navarra, R. J. (2011). Gottman method couple therapy: From theory to practice. In D. K. Carson & M. Casado-Kehoe (Eds.), *Case studies in couples therapy: Theory-based approaches* (pp. 331–343). Retrieved from http:// books.google.com.my.
Nurlaelawati, E. (2013). Muslim women in Indonesian religious courts: Reform, strategies, and pronouncement of divorce. *Islamic L. & Soc'y*, 20, 242.
Proulx, C. M., Helms, H. M., & Buehler, C. (2007). Marital quality and personal well-being: A meta-analysis. *Journal of Marriage and Family*, 69(3), 576–593.
Rakhshani, F., Niknami, S., & Ansari Moghadam, A. (2005). Couple communication in family planning decision-making in Zahedan. *Eastern Mediterranean Health Journal*, 11(4), 586–593.
Sadeghi, F. S., & Kalhor, S. (2007). Gap between genders in Iranian 3th development strategy. *Journal of Women* Studies, 2, 5–28.
Sanders, T. T. (2010). Premarital counseling: An assessment of the readiness of social workers to promote an approach to divorce prevention. (Doctoral dissertation). Retrieved from ProQuest. (3391590).
Sarookani, B. (2005). Women power and family. *Women Research*, 3(2), 29–50.
Schneider, I. (2016). Polygamy and legislation in contemporary Iran: An analysis of the public legal discourse. *Iranian Studies*, 49(4), 657–676.
Sillars, A., Canary, D. J., & Vangelisti, A. (2013). Conflict and relational quality in families. In A. L. Vangelisti (Ed.), *The Routledge handbook of family communication* (pp. 338–357). New York: Routledge.
Weeks, G. R., & Fife, S. T. (2014). *Couples in treatment: Techniques and approaches for effective practice*. New York: Routledge.
Woszidlo, A., & Segrin, C. (2013). Negative affectivity and educational attainment as predictors of newlyweds' problem solving communication and marital quality. *The Journal of Psychology, 147*(1), 49–73. doi:10.1080/00223980.2012.674069.

5

COUNSELING GREEK-CYPRIOT CLIENTS

Fotini Kranou Kyriakides

Introduction

The cultural group this chapter focuses on is clients of Cypriot descent, though information may be used for work with Greek clients due to cultural similarities between the two groups. This chapter provides background information regarding the family, social and cultural values, tradition, and financial issues that Cypriot clients face, as well as basic characteristics of their personality. It provides hands-on guidelines, specific step by step therapeutic interventions, techniques, and strategies, and recommendations based on theories derived from counseling and psychotherapy as well as from this writer's personal professional experience.

Cyprus is a European island located in the Eastern Mediterranean sea. Due to its geological location, Cyprus attracts a large number of foreign citizens for work, education, retirement, investment opportunities, and conflict zone refugees. Greek Cypriots and citizens of Greece share the same language and religion and related cultural traits and characteristics. The topic of the case study presented is this chapter examines family of origin which is a common issue when counseling Cypriot clients.

In order to be able to work on family independence issues with a client, as well as most clinical issues, a non-Cypriot counselor will need to be informed and enlightened about the Cypriot culture for therapy to be effective. Cypriot families maintain close and strong ties between their family members and parents, and continue to have close relationships with their families of origin even after marriage. Individuals hold strong social relationships with in-group members and are hesitant to accept and trust out-of-group individuals at the outset of meeting new people. Though a number of marriages between Cypriots and non-Cypriots take place, the majority of Cypriot individuals marry other Cypriots. Moreover, Cypriots are characterized by being highly religious and holding strong ties with their church of affiliation, which is Christian Orthodox. Major life events such as birth, marriage, and death are marked by traditional religious rituals (Killian & Agathangelou, 2005).

Family counselors working in Cyprus or abroad with Cypriot immigrants need to be aware that it was not easy for counseling (mental health) to become popular in Cyprus, mainly because for the fact that for decades individuals confided in their priests (Rollins, 2006) and sought advice from their teachers, or from older family members. Moreover, people did not view psychology and psychiatry as being two different fields, thus the client visiting a mental health professional viewed the self as "stigmatized" or "mentally ill." An important piece of information for counselors working with clients from Cyprus is that Cypriots do not express their feelings and emotions with ease, and they do so if and when they feel comfortable. Counseling and family counseling in Cyprus were not popular until after the 1990s as most mental health practitioners were clinical psychologists. Counselors and psychotherapists who studied in countries like the USA and Canada found it difficult to establish their professional identity and area of specialization.

There remains an increased need for continuing education in order to develop multicultural competence, counseling skills, and awareness in Cyprus. Another challenge addressed in this chapter is the lack of research discussing counseling with Cypriot or Greek families. The majority of counseling techniques books and manuals written by Cypriot or Greek theorists and therapists use Western European or American bibliographies which refersto specific techniques and practices primarily applicable to American and Western European clients. Family counseling literature on culturally competent treatment is limited for clients with Eastern European, Greek and Greek-Cypriot descent.

Family counselors are influenced by the conditioning of their particular cultural group. The cultural differences in shared assumptions and prescriptive rules sometimes lead to incongruent messages being given to families from a different culture. Some recurrent areas of difficulty in work with 'ethnic' families include the culture bound symptoms and family structures that do not conform to Western nuclear family norms (Lau, 1984). Moreover, there is no one single integrated therapeutic model for family counselors to rely on when working with clients from different cultures (Nichols & Shwarz, 2001).

Cypriot clients, as also clients from other cultures, view themselves from a "dual perspective." Norton's (1978) dual perspective holds that every individual is simultaneously embedded in at least two systems: that of the immediate nurturing physical (various elements in each particular culture and determines needs and sense of identity of the individual) and social environment, and that of the larger major society. Cypriot clients residing in Cyprus or abroad are proud of their ethnic identities and believe in connectedness. Ethnic identities are constructed within the context of "evolving products of material and social circumstances and the actions of the groups themselves, wrestling with, interpreting and responding to those circumstances, building or transforming (ethnic) identities in the process" (Cornell, 2000, p. 42). Connectedness is the recount of an ethnic group's collective cultural narratives further reflective of their ongoing interpretations of distinctive elements and linking together past, anticipated, and imagined experiences in a causal, sequential, and associational manner in a continuously changing world (Cornell, 2000).

This chapter, through theories derived from counseling and psychotherapy as well as from the author's personal practice experience, provide specific information for working more effectively with Cypriot families and couples. Moreover, it provides counselors with current background information regarding the family, social, culture and cultural values, tradition, and financial issues that Cypriot clients face, as well as characteristics of their cultural personality.

Cultural Competency with Cypriot Clients

> Culture is that set of shared world views, meanings, and adaptive behaviors derived from simultaneous membership and participation in a variety of contexts such as language; rural, urban, or suburban setting; race, ethnicity, and socioeconomic status; age, gender, religion, nationality; employment and occupation, political ideology, and stages of acculturation. (Falicov, 1983, pp. xiv–xv)

Pedersen (1991) states that multiculturism is the fourth force in psychology and Nieto (1992) holds that multiculturalism is based on the belief that all cultures have values, beliefs, and worldviews. Family counselors must be multiculturally competent when entering the counseling process and understand, as well as view, the case from the framework and environment of the personal culture of the client (Sue, Arrendondo & McDavis, 1994; Sue & Sue, 2007). Most counseling theories and practices are based on Western cultures and are developed and studied mainly by theorists and therapists in the United States of America and in Western Europe. The vast majority of the counseling theories refer to working with clients of Western descent, are not applied or tested for reliability or for effectiveness in various cultures and it is safe to say that applying counseling methods without modifying them to "fit" in a certain culture may have negative results in the counseling process. From 1973 to 2003 a majority of counseling and family therapy publications acknowledged the error of approaching family problems of ethnic minorities using the middle-class white American family as a frame of reference; theories in their majority fail to capture the complexity and adversity and as a result therapists are given a distorted homogenized caricature of other cultures leading them to the question of how much culture tailoring they need to do in their daily clinical practice (Ho et al., 2004).

Culturally competent counseling can take place only when the cultural contributions of all parties in the counseling process are explored (Tyler et al., 1991). A culturally attuned therapist must understand the ethnic themes in a family's history and take a stance for it as understanding ethnic themes will help the counselor to uncover the family's narrative world; a counselor cannot understand a family's problem if without recognizing the material and elements of the predominant sociocultural metanarratives and the role they play in the individual's experiences (Ho et al., 2004).

For example, the author is a Cypriot counselor who was educated in Louisiana, USA in a Master's Degree Counseling Program. During her program of study, she worked with a wide range of issues with American clients at the university's counseling center, with Vietnam veterans at a Veteran's Administration Center, and with incarcerated males at a correctional facility in Louisiana. When she begun working with Cypriot clients upon her return to Cyprus, it became obvious that some of the counseling theories, practices, and techniques utilized in the USA needed to be modified to better fit the needs of the Cypriot clientele. Though clinical symptoms, diagnosis, and theories in their general and basic forms are common and apply to clients from most cultures, the techniques, approach, setting of boundaries and therapy goals needed some revision and adaptation.

Case Examples

The two following case illustrations are to lead to a better understanding by comparing two case studies of clients of different decent.

Case Study One: "Erin"

Erin, an American individual 18 years of age from Monroe, Louisiana needing to feel and become more independent from her family came to the author's office in the USA seeking counseling. She had received family counseling for three months when she was 12 and her mother was pregnant with her second sister. Therefore, she knew what to expect during the process.

Erin's Case Illustration

Erin was familiar with the counseling process and felt comfortable initiating the contact.	Erin called the counseling office and arranged an appointment for herself.
This author, as a foreign trainee counselor, had adequate information and training (both theoretical and clinical) on how to work with American clients. As an individual, she had to understand, respect, and become more familiar with the differences of Erin's culture as compared to her culture (Cypriot families pay for their children's higher education), provide with accommodation, transportation and spending money. Furthermore, this author needed to understand the difference between the two cultures as at that time (late 1990s), 18-year-old females in her country did not live alone unless they were at the university, it was not common to support themselves financially, and the majority were not allowed to stay with their boyfriend.	Erin worked at a local department store and bought her car with money she earned herself. Her salary was low so she could not rent her own apartment. On the weekends she stayed with her boyfriend in Shreveport. Her family approved of her relationship with her boyfriend. Furthermore, her family was supportive of her, accepting her lifestyle and letting her choose whether she would become further educated or not.

(Continued)

(Cont.)

Implication for close mother-daughter dyadic relationship, sister-two younger siblings' triadic relationship. Counselor and client discussed various relationships in the immediate family and these were explored further in a genogram.	Erin complained that her family home was loud as she had three younger siblings and that she was usually asked to help with chores like babysitting and grocery shopping. This usually led to arguments and sometimes fights between her and her parents and her and her siblings. She also felt close to them and felt guilty for wanting to leave the family nest.
Family system boundary was threatened.	She also felt guilty for "leaving" her mother alone with her father as the couple had marital problems. Erin usually defended or emotionally protected and parented her mother.
Triangulation case: family conflict led to physical and psychological symptoms.	Erin, caught in the middle, developed a mild eating disorder and mild depressive symptomatology.
Erin had the opportunity to talk and be understood in a safe and understanding environment. She was relieved. She felt hope for the future.	In the sessions that followed, counselor and client discussed feelings, her role in the nuclear family, the stress and burden she felt, the depressive and eating disorder symptoms, homework was given and more therapy goals were discussed.
Negotiating and stabilizing the new family structure.	Her parents had an appointment alone with the therapist in order to discuss Erin's feelings. They were asked if they knew Erin felt this way about her role in their relationship, if they had suggestions and the need for roles to be redefined in the family system was discussed.
Individual sessions to achieve self- understanding and empowerment and to enhance her transactions with her family.	In the following months counselor and client had weekly sessions with Erin in order to discuss the previously mentioned issues. Moreover, the means of her becoming more independent (i.e., finding a job with a higher salary, receiving university education or education at a training center, saving for rental money to move out of her home, better scheduling of her own program) were discussed.

(Continued)

(Cont.)

Towards the end of the six-month cooperation, Erin was encouraged to build herself around her independence, emotional, educational and social needs.	Erin applied to study computer engineering at the university and decided to continue working at the department store to save for rental and personal expense money. She decided to move out of the house and rent a one-bedroom apartment in southern Monroe, which was cheaper and closer to work. She would visit her family during the week for dinner.

Case Study Two: "Marina"

Marina, a Cypriot 18-year-old individual wishing to work on her independence from her family came hesitantly to my office in Cyprus. She was referred to the author by her family physician as he believed that Marina's frequent headaches and weight gain were caused by high levels of stress, general dissatisfaction, by the fact that she failed classes in the university program she was enrolled in, and argued often with her parents.

Marina's Case Illustration

Counseling is new to Marina.	Marina only told her mother about her wish to go to counseling, but no one else.
The counselor, being Cypriot and from the same culture, understood how she felt. Counseling is still stigmatized in a few rural communities. In these communities and in a very small percentage of people living in the cities, people receiving mental health counseling are viewed as weak, with "problematic behavior," or with psychiatric problems. A common comment of individuals of this small sub-culture is "Why would I go to a counselor? I am not crazy" or "Why would I take my child to a counselor? My child is strong, smart and definitely not crazy."	Marina was shy at first and did not talk a lot, nor maintained eye contact with the counselor.
Due to the cities' smaller size compared to larger cities in Europe and the USA, it is common for counselors to know socially the client's family and social environment. It is not uncommon for this author's clients to ask if she would leave an empty space of a few minutes before and after their session, especially if they are more well-known to the community.	During the first session, confidentiality issues were explained as she was worried about the possibility of me knowing her father or other relatives.

(Continued)

(Cont.)

The client felt comfortable and understood. The counselor asked what the issues that brought her to the office are, and what she feels she would need to work on.	Marina feels like she needs to "grow up" and live alone. Her university is in her hometown, therefore she lives with her parents. She drives her car to class, which was a graduation gift from her parents.
The counselor understands that in Cyprus, it is still believed by many families that girls should live with their parents until they get married, unless they study or work in a different city or abroad. The "clean cut" image of a single girl is considered crucial for her status in society. A counselor from a different culture could have asked "Why don't you find a job, save up and move out of the house?" This would not be applicable in this case without conflict between the family members.	Marina does not need to explain in detail why her family does not let her live alone. She feels understood.
University education is not a matter of a personal decision for a large percentage of young individuals as it is expected that they *will* enter a university program upon high school graduation. Only a small percentage of individuals does not apply or receive university or college education. Moreover, if there is a family business which is successful, the children usually continue working for it and study in a relevant field.	Marina's father is a successful accountant leading his own firm with more than 30 employees. He wishes that his daughter will graduate in accounting and join him as a junior partner in the firm. Marina wanted to study fine arts at a university in another city. Her father wishes for her to earn high income and believes that fine art studies and activities are something she can view as a hobby. Both paternal and maternal grandparents shared her father's view.
Here is a culturally sensitive approach to Marina's case. When this author worked with this particular client, she emphasized relationships with maternal and paternal families of origin. Extended family has a significant role in decision-making for their married children and their grandchildren.	Counselor and client discussed the possibility of the father being informed of the sessions and her talking to him about her wish to study fine arts. In the genogram, the relationships between the parents, between parents and Marina, Marina and siblings, Marina, her parents and paternal and maternal grandparents clarified more details.
If a counselor with no adequate knowledge of the Cypriot culture were to work with the father, she could have thought of the father as being strict, non-respectful to his daughter's feelings, authoritative, etc.	Marina's father joined the counseling process in the fifth session. He initially asked the counselor jokingly if his beliefs are "problematic." It was understood that behind his joke, he felt uncomfortable to be in the session.

(Continued)

(Cont.)

	During that discussion, information about his upbringing was asked. He was born and raised in a rural area of the island in a small village of about 500 inhabitants. His parents were poor farmers who worked 13 hour days and saved enough money to buy property in areas that gained high value today. When he graduated from high school, his parents told him that he could either help them in the farm and fields or enroll in a university. They told him that in order for them to pay for his education with their hard earned money, he could study in one of the following areas: medicine, law, or accounting. He met his wife at the university while she was studying law. She started her successful practice and works full time up to today. Their three children were raised with much help of the grandparents. His parents moved in with them in a semi-attached condo to their house to help babysit the children,
During the discussion, it was clear that the father's upbringing and his relationship with his parents influenced his relationship with his children and his expectations from them.	He realized that he became much like his father. He still wanted his daughter to study in a prosperous field and be financially well-off, but he also remembered that he wanted to study philosophy as a young adult. He agreed to think further and discuss the probability of his daughter studying fine arts or graphic arts.
Self-disclosure gains appreciation and respect towards the counselor in the Cypriot culture thus leading the client to feel more comfortable, as well as view the counselor as a simple individual with similar concerns to theirs.	The counselor expressed understanding and respect towards the family values and disclosed that she herself started her studies in the pre-elementary education field and switched her degree to psychology in the second year after discussing it with her family. Both father and daughter appreciated her disclosure.

The counselor's personal values and beliefs should not override those of the clients; only after the intercultural viewpoints are understood can the counselor continue to assess the behavior accurately and to advocate changes properly (Locke, 1998). Therefore, if Marina were to seek counseling from a counselor who had no knowledge of her descent background, culture, social traits, and who used mainstream techniques and practices, the result might have proved to be negative. It could help the individual become more independent for a period of time, but it could also mean that she would become estranged from her family of origin.

Counselors should be careful when they develop assumptions and agendas during the counseling process when working with clients from a culture other than their own. On the other hand, they should not over-attribute symptoms and dysfunctions to the client's culture. For family and couple counseling to be successful with Cypriot clients and clients from different cultures the following guided practice steps will assist the counselors (Celano & Kaslow, 2000):

1. The counselor must understand the effect his or her own culture has on the therapeutic relationship.
2. Recognize that the theories and techniques of choice reflect the culture within which they have been developed.
3. Appreciate the dynamic interplay of the cultural influences affecting the client and his or her family's functioning.
4. Develop and implement culturally acceptable problem-resolution strategies.

Counselors should bear in mind the following when working with Cypriot individuals and families:

1. Older Cypriot clients are hesitant to come to the first sessions out of worry that "someone else will find out."
2. Older clients view their need to receive counseling as a sign of weakness.
3. During the initial session, the counselor should explain:

    a. The counselor should state the name and credentials, area of training, a few sentences regarding the type of therapy that will be used. It is not uncommon for clients to ask where the counselor studied and how many years of practice they had, therefore a non-Cypriot counselor should not be offended. Handshakes are common to take place at the beginning and end of the initial session.
    b. Confidentiality issues. It is more usual rather than rare for clients to see friends and relatives in the waiting room or at the entrance. It is also usual that the counselor and the client have people they know in common. Moreover, it is probable that the counselor sees other family members or classmates of the client. If the Cypriot client does not trust the counselor during the first session, they will not come back. Cypriot parents and

children have close relationships. Moreover, young adults of the age of 18 are still considered children by the majority of the parents. The counselor should place strict boundaries with the parents regarding the information given in a session between the counselor and their child.

Setting Boundaries for Therapy

Cyprus is a small country with villages and small cities. It is probable that the client and the counselor share common friends, relatives, neighbors, etc. The counselor should clearly state that questions and comments regarding the people they know in common are strictly forbidden.

The fact that the counselor and the client might have common social acquaintances, might lead the client to view the counselor as a friend. The counselor can be friendly during therapy, but explain the difference between the possible friendly approach and kind personality and the fact that they are not and cannot be friends.

During the therapeutic procedure of counselors working with Cypriot individuals and families, the following guidelines and cultural information will be of assistance:

1. Goal-setting between the counselor and the client must take into consideration cultural concerns, like the role of authority, the process of decision-making, perceptions of the etiology and meaning attribution to family problems and their solutions, and the cultural viewpoints of both the client and the counselor (Celano & Kaslow, 2000); (Kaslow et al., 1995; 1998).
2. The counselor joining the individual or the family is crucial in forming and developing a working alliance and this can be adapted to the client's and the counselor's cultural context, as well to the co-created cultural context between the client and the counselor (Szapocznic et al., 1997). "To some extent, the ways in which the therapist allies with the family is dependent upon whether she/he is identified as a member of the family's cultural group. While the importance of the therapist-client cultural matching is controversial, cultural matching is probably a distal rather than proximal factor affecting treatment response" (Celano & Kaslow, 2000, p. 222).
3. Open-ended questions that expect disclosures to take place, or reflecting feelings and emotions may not be productive; clients from Cyprus tend to keep information to themselves and find it difficult to self-disclose (Danielidou & Hovarth, 2006).
4. This does not mean that feelings and emotions are not significant in the counseling process; an environment of openness and trust among the family system is developed from preliminary insights and data that help the system understand what will help the counseling process (Zagelbaum & Carlson, 2011).

5. Referring to Cypriot clients, Zagelbaum and Carlson state that "family systems can trust the counseling process to locate strengths and engage family members in a forward-focused process whereby goals can be reassessed and revisited during each session to determine where process has been made. The process of the family counseling is aided by the progress of the system" (p. 206).
6. A culturally competent counselor will understand that the Greek culture is mainly patriarchal. The father figure is highly respected and viewed as the main financial supporter of the family. Historically and in the recent past, the man's authority was rarely questioned, whereas the females were traditionally expected to support their husbands on all matters (Killian & Agathangelou, 2005).
7. A counselor working with adults or children of Cypriot origin needs to apprehend what is frequently mentioned in this chapter: parent and child relationships are very important in the Cypriot family system across all ages and stages of the client's life span. The statement by Papajohn and Spiegel (1975) still remains true to this day: "Generational separations are sharp, and a son in his 40s relates to his father with the same manifestations of respect expected of him as a child" (p. 182). Parents are loving and protecting of their sons and daughters and at the same time strict. Children are expected to act within the social norms, behave, and represent the family's clean image in various social settings (school, family and social gatherings).
8. Parent and children relationships affect almost all areas of the children's decision-making, including higher education and career choice. Parents have high expectations regarding their children's studies and university of choice. College education, choice of study and choice of university is usually a stressful matter in the Cypriot families with parents and children disagreeing on the area of study.
9. Marital and relationship issues are similar to those of the European and Western world, therefore this chapter will not discuss them in detail. The one marital issue that is prevalent, though, and may not be present in many other cultures, is the involvement of the maternal and paternal family of origin in the new couple's married life. This was very common in the past decades and still present in a number of today's couples.
10. The involvement of the family of origin includes grandparents, parents, and siblings of the new husband and wife. Some issues that cause marital conflict include:

    i. Financial handling issues: In some systems, the family of origin is aware of the financial situation of the couple, agrees or disagrees with the couple's expenses and may have a strong standpoint in the couple's financial decisions. The counselor can assist the couple by providing them with encouragement to explore the ways to how better manage their financial issues, advising them to speak to a financial consultant if they need to, guide them to ask themselves if their parents' involvement in their monetary matters is important and very importantly assist them in trusting each other as they trust their parents.

ii. Children's upbringing: In a number of families, grandparents of both sides might attempt to interfere and influence the way children are raised because usually grandparents of both sides are the care takers of the children for the hours that the parents work. Therefore, the assistance provides the grandparents with the role of the "Assistant parent." This in turn gives the grandparents "access" to the area of the child's upbringing.

iii. Location of the living arrangements of the couple: In older years, the bride's family would build or buy a house as a gift to the couple as close as possible to the maternal family. If the couple chose to stay far away, it could mean disrespect or aversion of the new spouse towards his or her in laws. This is not as customary in the past 20 years.

iv. Naming of the children. In the past, it was customary that the first son would be named after the paternal grandfather to continue the family name (similar to USA couples naming a son after the father and adding Jr. after the name). It was also customary to name the first daughter after the maternal grandmother. In present times the couple names their child with a personal name of choice or after their parents only if *they* wish to do so.

The counselor should create a genogram and ask specific questions as per the role that the maternal and paternal grandparents, uncles and aunts play in the daily life of the nuclear family, as well as the roles up taken by older siblings. Counselors may request to have a few sessions with the couple's parents separately. Moreover, the culturally accustomed counselor may view the individual, the couple and the children in terms of the ecosystem framework which emphasizes the "person-in-environment" point of view understanding the unique experiences of each population.

> An ecosystem framework provides a lens in which the family and family members can be understood within the context of transactions with a variety of biological, psychological, cultural, and historical environments. By adopting an ecosystem perspective, a family therapist can focus on adaptive (and maladaptive) transactions between the persons and various environments, that is, the interface between them. (Ho et al., 2004, p. 11)

There might exist several ecological contexts where a counselor would be asked to discover the family's culture and its ecological niche (Falicov, 1998).

When counseling couples in Cyprus, the counselor will work mostly with intermarried couples (both being Cypriot, Christian Orthodox, and share the same culture). It is important for a counselor to discern that in the past (early 19th century), the patriarchal Cypriot family model left little decision-making to the females of the household, whereas sons were to continue the family name, business, heritage, and financial success. It was more common for sons to become further educated after high school and for daughters to marry and have children. This has gradually changed in the last 50 years with couples having approached a more Western gender role model. As in most cultures, both genders work, share household expenses, study locally or abroad, sons and daughters have equal positions in the family and equal educational or job opportunities. When discussing pre-divorce or post-divorce relationships, as well as when working with children of divorced parents, the counselor must keep in mind that divorce is a major stigma in the Cypriot and Greek culture (Killian & Agathangelou, 2005). As in most other cultures, older siblings develop a "guardian," "second-parent," or a "supporter" role in order to assist and attempt to ease the pain of younger siblings or the hurt parent that stayed behind. This might subsequently lead to this sibling's emotional burnout with the result of probable depressive symptoms, interpersonal and intrapersonal issues, lack of interest in age appropriate activities, and a decrease of school grades.

Cases of individuals with depression and stress disorder (with growing incidents of panic attack episodes) visiting counselors increased during and after March 2013 up to today as a result of the colossal financial crisis in the March 2013 that left banks closed for days and led to a haircut of personal and business bank accounts that caused Cypriots to lose millions of euros and property. Savings of a lifetime disappeared overnight, businesses closed down leaving urban areas deserted. The large unemployment rate caused a series of new to Cyprus social phenomena like receiving food items from church stores for free and free breakfast for a large number of students at school. Some brought their families with them at some stage and some went alone leaving behind their wives and children. It also caused something quite unexpected: there were no riots, no fights, no stealing, and no ethical collapse. Strangers helped strangers and people stoically abided the rules imposed by the International Monetary Fund (i.e., for months there was only a limited amount of money people were allowed to receive from ATMs). Families, friends and colleagues came closer and there was a sense of pride in people's behavior.

The financial crisis in Cyprus affected individuals to the extent of restricting visits to counselors or even their private physicians due to cost. NGOs, the church, and other charity organizations understood the need of counseling being available for free, or for a minimal fee, and arranged for therapists to provide help. Counselors were also affected by the financial crisis. A large number of their clients had to immediately terminate therapy, break for a period of time, or minimize the number of sessions (for example instead of weekly sessions, the clients could afford monthly sessions).

A counselor working with a Cypriot affected by this crisis should become informed about the history and effects on economy and society before the initial session. Due to the subject's sensitivity, as well as it being so recent, the client might cry, express feelings of anger, shame, and guilt. The counselor needs to let the client express their feelings and express sympathy. Their feelings need to be heard, understood and though the client needs to feel comfort, a counselor's comment like "*I understand that you feel hurt and fear at this present stage of your life, but you have your whole life ahead of you and blank pages of your book to write in as the author of your life*" could make the client uncomfortable, not understood, even angry. This category of client comes to counseling to essentially grieve and the steps and treatment goals should include similar work and approach as in grief and mourning therapy. It is imperative that feelings like shock, anger, and sadness are discussed as it is significant that issues like self-actualization, self-esteem, motivation, plans for the future, and family relationships are explored.

Conclusions and Recommendations

Further practical guidelines following are adapted by Zagelbaum and Carlson (2011) and are presented here as useful techniques when working with Cypriot clients:

1. Unceasingly seek training in cultural competence.
2. Adopt a culturally humble approach.
3. Use culturally appropriate tools.
4. Examine the client's worldview on wellness, religion and the role of faith in wellness.
5. Provide culturally competent preventive psychoeducation.

As explained in detail, a significant number of the Cypriot clients are skeptical of mental health services. Attrition will take place if the counselor does not understand the client's culture, history, family circumstances or fails to join her/him and the family and if alliance is not formed. Two proximal variables that will enhance the counseling process and client-counselor relationship are giving and credibility (Sue & Zane, 1987). Giving is an important variable that might help the client trust and ally with the counselor and it refers to providing the family with a direct benefit of therapy early in the treatment. Credibility refers to the ascribed status of the counselor by the client or the client's family or a status achieved through demonstrated skills and culturally competent interventions through which the counselor will gain the client's trust both as a person and as a professional. A competent counselor should frequently revisit the approaches taken with clients from different cultures and continuously educate the self with information about the history, politics, social issues and cultural and ethnic characteristics of individuals from other cultures visiting her/his office. Failure to incorporate cultural perspectives might lead the counselors to adopting unproductive methodologies in their attempt to work with the client. Understanding multicultural issues in counseling will provide more sensitive, competent and effective approaches in terms of relating to the client and the client's issues.

References

Celano, M., & Kaslow, N. (2000). Culturally competent family interventions: Review and case illustrations. *The American Journal of Family Therapy*, 28, 217–228.

Cornell, S. (2000). That's the story of our life. In P. R. Spickard & W. J. Burroughs (Eds.), *Narrative and multiplicity in constructing ethnic identities* (pp. 41–53). Philadelphia, PA: Temple University Press.

Danielidou, L., & Hovarth, P. (2006). Greek Cypriot attitudes toward Turkish Cypriots and Turkish immigrants. *Journal of Social Psychology*, 146, 405–421.

Falicov, C. J. (Ed.). (1983). *Cultural perspectives in family therapy*. Rockville, MD: Aspen.

Falicov, C. J. (1998). *Latino families in therapy*. New York: Guilford Press.

Ho, M. K., Matthews-Rasheed, J., & Rasheed, M. N. (2004). *Family therapy with ethnic minorities*. Newbury Park, CA: Sage Publications.

Kaslow, N. J., Celano, M., & Dreelin, E. D. (1995). A cultural perspective on family theory and therapy. *Psychiatric Clinics of North America*, 18, 621–633.

Kaslow, N. J., Loundy, M., & Wood, K. (1998). A cultural perspective on families across the life-cycle: Family patterns, assessment, and intervention. In A. S. Bellack & M. Hersen (Eds.), *Comprehensive clinical psychology* (pp. 173–205). New York: Pergamon Press.

Killian, K. D., & Agathangelou, A. (2005). Greek families. In M. McGoldrick, J. Giordano, & J. Garcia-Preto (Eds.), *Ethnicity and family therapy* (pp. 573–585). New York: Guilford Press.

Lau, A. (1984). Transcultural issues in family therapy. *Journal of Family Therapy*, 6, 91–112.

Locke, D. C. (1998). *Increasing Multicultural Understanding: A Comprehensive Model* (2nd ed.). London: Sage.

Nichols, M., & Schwartz, R. (2001). *Essentials in family therapy*. New York: Allyn & Bacon.

Nieto, S. (1992). *Affirming diversity: The sociopolitical context of multicultural education*. New York: Longman.

Norton, D. G. (1978). *The dual perspective: Inclusion of ethnic minority content in the social work curriculum*. New York: Council on Social Work Education.

Papajohn, J., & Spiegel, J. (1975). *Transactions in families*. New York: Jossey-Bass.

Pedersen, P. B. (1991). Multiculturalism as a generic approach to counseling. *Journal of Counseling & Development*, 70, 6–12.

Rollins, J. (2006). Getting a global perspective: A glimpse of the counseling profession in 27 countries. *Counseling Today*, 1, 1–34.

Sue, D. W., & Sue, D. (2007). *Counseling the culturally different: Theory and practice* (5th ed.). New York: Wiley.

Sue, D. W., Arredondo, P., & McDavis, R. J. (1994). Multicultural counseling competencies and standards: A call to the profession. *Journal of Counseling and Development*, 70, 477–486.

Sue, S., & Zane, N. (1987). The role of culture and cultural techniques in psycho-therapy: A critique and reformulation. *American Psychologist*, 42(1), 37–45.

Tyler, F. B., Brome, D. R., & Williams, J. E. (1991). *Ethnic validity, ecology, and psychotherapy: A psychological competence model*. New York: Plenum Press.
Szapocznik, J., Kurtines, W. M., Santisteban, D., Pantin, H., Scopetta, M., Mancilla, Y., Aisenberg, S., McIntosh, S., Perez-Vidal, A., & Coatsworth, J. D. (1997). The evolution of structural ecosystemic theory for working with Latino families. In J. G. Garcia & M. C. Zea (Eds.), *Psychological interventions and research with Latino populations* (pp. 166–190). Boston, MA: Allyn & Bacon.
Zagelbaum, J., & Carlson, A. (2011). *Working with immigrant families: A practical guide for counselors*. New York: Routledge.

Additional Resources

Gari, A., & Kalantzi-Azizi, A. (1998). The influence of traditional values of education on Greek students' real and ideal self-concepts. *The Journal of Social Psychology*, 138(1), 5–12, doi:10.1080/00224549809600348.

6

COUPLE COUNSELING IN TURKEY

Considering Relationship Beliefs and Gender Roles

Berke Kirikkanat

Introduction

Family counseling is a broad framework which generally aims at facilitating interpersonal relationships within the family by focusing on the communication and relationship patterns among the family members. Turkey, representing a collectivistic structure in its family formations, has an increasing number of divorce as well as relationship break-ups. Turkish Statistical Institute (TUIK) reported in March 2016 that the number of the divorced people went up to 0.7% while the number of the married people rose to 0.5%, compared to the previous year. Being misunderstood is one of the most crucial factors why the couples conflict with each other harshly. Especially, the couples' beliefs about what is right and wrong in a romantic relationship, who is the ideal partner to be married, what is to be expected from a romantic partner etc. and their gender roles are greatly shaped by their cultural background. These issues have a pivotal impact on their marital adjustment and satisfaction. Thus, this chapter will consider the possible effects of dysfunctional relationship beliefs and traditional gender roles of Turkish couples on the quality of their romantic relationships. It will also cover the basic practical implications which can be useful for studying with Turkish couples.

Many people worry about whether he or she can find the true love in his or her life and be with the most loveable person throughout life. During this journey, a person may experience painful feelings and disappointments as he thinks that his partner does not have the expected qualities. Why do we have such criteria for our possible partners in a romantic relationship? Where do these ideas derive from? How do our perceptions about romantic attachments, marriages, or family lives shape our close relationships and the potential conflicts in them?

These questions bring us to those days when love is discussed very profoundly with the mythological figures. For Plato, in his well-known *Symposium*, human being suffers from the search for their soulmate throughout his life due to the harsh treatment of Zeus, the God of the gods in Greek mythology (Jowett & Pelliccia, 1996). Plato states that in those years, humankind is formed in three different types who have four legs, four arms and a head with two facial sides: man–man, woman–woman, and man–woman. As they increase in numbers, they think they can fight against gods and become the most powerful entity in the world. Zeus recognized such an arrogant attitude in his creatures and punished them by drifting apart all of them into two components and sending them to the other side of the earth (Jowett & Pelliccia, 1996). Because of this rough punishment, we, all have the drive to explore the possible partner options in our romantic acquaintances.

Regan (2011) claims that there are three pivotal requirements in which two people fulfill so as to make them think that they are involved in a relationship: 1) there must be a reciprocal impact between the two (one's emotional or behavioral attitude affects the other one's feelings or deeds as well); 2) their mutual companionship must have inimitable characteristics which are distinguished from the usual interaction with the other people in the society; 3) based on the communication, each side must have a mental framework of their affair. To Regan (2011), a close relationship between two individuals can be seen as mating, friendship, or family union. These relationships are complicated in nature, which are embedded by the systems containing physical circumstances (e.g., the weather conditions, geographical position etc.), social circumstances (e.g., neighbors, family members etc.), society (e.g., the country in which relationship takes place) and culture (e.g., individualistic or collectivistic cultures etc.) Therefore, an intimate companionship includes not only two individuals having unique cognitive, emotional, and behavioral repertoire but also the larger psychosocial and cultural conditions. In order to examine the quality of romantic relations in a couple who apply to marriage and family counseling to enhance their relationship satisfaction, one must take into consideration both the relationship schemas / beliefs of the couple and the gender roles shaping their minds since their childhood.

Dysfunctional Relationship Beliefs

Individuals have different perceptions regarding romantic relationships (courtship, marriage etc.). Perceptions in romantic bonds are related to the ways of comprehending the interplays with the loved one in the relationship (Dattilio, 2010). These perceptions are composed of the schemas pertinent to emotional exchanges. Schemas are depicted as the theoretical frameworks of how social life functions (Chen, 2001). Schemas are the tools of organizing one's interpretative world in a unique manner (Kelly, 1955). They help us survive from information overloaded and facilitate reaching a conclusion on a topic easily. Schemas about relationships, on the other hand, include how we describe our partners and communications in our minds. They play a critical role on forming our relationship structures with our partners.

Relationship schemas can be depicted as cognitive shortcuts used to shape one's relational interactions (Baldwin, 1992). They are constituted based on prior experiences shaped by family of origin and conventional rules in the society where one is raised, and initial emotional contacts in childhood, adolescence and early adulthood (Dattilio, 2010). They consist of three components (Baldwin, 1992): a script displaying a series of events in which two partners behave, feel, or think in a relationship; a self-schema; and a schema for the other one in which each partner has a mental framework about himself or herself and each other in a relational domain. To Baldwin (1992), the first two components are associated with the concepts called self-perception and impression formation. On the other hand, the relational script is a new point to be focused, which directs one's relationship future.

To Fiske and Haslam (1996), individuals have different cognitive relational models which can be categorized based on the four elements: "communal sharing, equality matching, authority ranking and market pricing" (Fiske & Haslam, 1996, p. 144). The ones forming their relations in reference to communal sharing pay an extensive attention to the prevalent features between them. Especially, they look at their similarities rather than their differences, which in turn leads to a homogeneous relation between the two. Nationality, ethnicity, and religion are critical terms used for appreciating potential partner preferences. Another element utilized by partners is equality matching in which both of them establish their interactional patterns in an equitable and redeeming fashion. Those individuals try to create a harmony in the relationship. Authority ranking, on the other hand, is another element leading to relationship formation based on one's social status or title. There is always a power imbalance in those relations. The last element pertinent to the cognitive relational models is market pricing. This concept leads the two to account the advantages and disadvantages of their partners as well as their relationships. Market pricing is directly associated with social exchange theory, which describes the fact that we prefer the ones who provide lots of benefits with very minimum costs (Thibaut & Kelley, 1959). It states that we try to decide whether to stay in our present romantic relationship or terminate it based on the degree of the profits we gain from that relationship.

For Knee (1998), individuals have different implicit theoretical frameworks about romantic relationships. These theories include one's beliefs regarding to how a relationship works. They contain one's thinking patterns regarding the essential ingredients of a good romantic partnership. According to Knee (1998), there are two kinds of beliefs molding future bonds: destiny belief and growth belief. The partners having a destiny belief are the ones who contemplate the degree of harmony in the relationship as a determinant factor for a successful bond. They try to analyze their relations in terms of the frequency of problems and dissatisfaction at the beginning of the relationship. If this frequency is high, they attempt to end the relationship as they think that such a beginning is a sign for a bad commitment in the future and no effort can heal this relation effectively. On the other hand, the partners having a growth belief are the ones who have the opinion that despite the handicaps in the relationship, it is worth to fight against them. They believe that the purpose of a relationship is to develop oneself and each other in the face of obstacles and cultivate the relationship in a constructive manner. Thus, growth belief makes romantic partners survive and keep their relations last longer than destiny belief.

Several researchers (Baucom, Epstein, Sayers, & Sher, 1989; Epstein & Eidelson, 1981; Filipovic, Vukosavljevic-Gvozden, & Opacic, 2016; Fincham & Bradbury, 1989; Gizir, 2013; Holmes, 2004; Kayser & Himle, 1994; Kurdek, 1993) try to address how the irrational thought patterns of couples damage the romantic partnership very profoundly. They state that these dysfunctional relationship beliefs cause the one to explain the other one's feelings, behaviors, and thoughts in an unrealistic manner. These irrational beliefs are derived from cognitive distortions made during emotional interaction with the romantic partner. Cognitive distortions include impractical ingredients of thoughts leading to lots of misunderstandings and erroneous perceptions about that person (Beck, 1963).

The irrational romantic beliefs deriving from the cognitive errors lead to several relational conflicts between couples. Here are the problems common in Turkey.

Any Argument in a Relationship Leads to its Termination

Such an idea makes partners avoid talking about their problems and expressing their feelings pertinent to the relational handicaps honestly. For example, as a couple counselor, I recognize that many couples prefer not having an argument with their partners in order to show their social networks such as their families, close friends, colleagues etc. that they have a perfect relationship and anyone or any event can harm this bond. Some couples state that they grew up in families where there were lots of escalating conflicts and nobody in the family had an attempt to solve these problems. In that way, they learned the avoidance coping strategy in their childhood as a means of protecting their relationship. It can be stated that couples learn the ways of ignoring the challenging situations in close relations from their past experiences with their parents, families etc.

Nonverbal Language between the Partners Is the Key for Ultimate Intimacy

This thought causes partners to feel disappointed when one partner does not have the ability to comprehend the other's feelings, thoughts, or behaviors by not using verbal language. The inability to read one's mind is seen as the lack of true love in the relationship. In Turkey, as Hamamcı (2005) found in her study, women place more value on mind reading in their relations than men. If this is not met by their partners, women feel frustrated and think that "He is not ideal for me!" Men, on the other hand, talk about their relational needs directly and do not have any attempt to use indirect messages to their partners. As I recognized in couple counseling, men usually complain about why their romantic partners do not tell their actual feelings to them straightforwardly and why women make all things complicated for them.

Being Very Intimate in a Romantic Relationship Makes the One Very Vulnerable to Physically and Mentally Arduous Feelings

An individual who usually thinks that being very close to his romantic partner opens the gates of vulnerability in his life has lots of attempts to look for high social distance toward his partner. Such an idea is based on the cognitive errors including mind reading and overgeneralization (Kayser & Himle, 1994). It includes avoidance from possible agonizing feelings in the relationship. The reason behind this behavior varies from previous hurtful experiences in childhood such as divorce, loss of a loved one, abandonment by someone very close to him, to gender roles in the society.

The impact of one's upsetting childhood experiences on the formation of dysfunctional attachment schemas is critically analyzed by Young, Klosko, and Weishaar (2003). They state that the people who have abandonment schema are afraid of being walked away from them by their loved ones through severe diseases, divorce, etc. While some of them display avoidant behaviors toward their romantic partners, some of them manifest high levels of dependency on their partners via very protective and jealous behaviors.

In my counseling sessions, I encounter a common problem in couples that they are like control-freak units who show overreliance on their partners by text-messaging, recording lots of pictures and videos and sending them to their companions immediately. They want their partners to understand "I am not cheating you and I am in love with you, you will not lose me anymore." When one of them does not fulfill such an expectation, harsh arguments between couples occur and high levels of frustration, anxiety, and disappointment are revealed. And if an actual loss of a partner arises, severe psychological disturbances such as major depression, bipolar disorder, panic attack, commitment phobia, and so on.

Another problem I would like to point out is that some males have more tendencies not to show their affection toward their partners than women due to the traditional gender roles prescribed in Turkish culture. Especially, men who are raised in families where having emotional deadness in social relations is necessary for being very powerful and dominant in the eyes of others in the society state that displaying their emotional sides makes them defenseless toward others. They assume that if they express their emotional components of personality, they will lose their authority in social network.

Doing Whatever the Other Partner Wants Is the Key for Successful Relationships

An individual who has an idea that the approval of the loved one guarantees his or her commitment to the relationship inclines to satisfy all physical and psychological needs of his or her partner. To Horney (1937), such a tendency derives from one's childhood experiences with his parents. Especially, how parents deal with their child's prevalent sense of loneliness and helplessness (e.g. basic anxiety) felt in infancy and how the child finds a way to handle with this anxiety are the key determinants of his personality. During this process, the child develops neurotic needs (e.g. unreasonable defense mechanisms against this anxiety) such as a desire to obtain emotional devotion and sanction, to have a preeminent companion, to attain success, etc. For Horney (1945), the two neurotic needs – acquiring strong fondness and approval, and having a predominant partner – are responsible for the development of compliant personality in the individual. The ones having such a personality are very sensitive to their partners' physical and psychological needs, and they tend to please them all the time and discount their own desires for the sake of the relationship.

On the other hand, to Gestalt perspective, such a belief results from the inability to have a meaningful relationship with natural and interpersonal world (e.g., contact). Specifically, the contact boundary problem called confluence is the main reason behind doing whatever the other partner wants (Polster & Polster, 1973). These individuals cannot say "No!" to their partners and express their own preferences to them straightforwardly. Instead of displaying their true feelings and thoughts, they always comply with their partners' wishes.

Young et al. (2003) explains the same belief via the concept called subjugation schema. To these researchers, the people having subjugation schema behave in a way of gratifying the others' needs and restraining their own needs in order to avert from their punishments, revenges, or feelings of anger. They forgo their own selves because they believe that if they make an attempt to tell their own desires to their partners, they will encounter harsh vengeance from their companions.

Among Turkish couples, it is recognized that women are in the role of self-sacrifice for the sake of successful relationship with their partners while men are in the role of dominant companion who both control and demand many things from their partners. When women understand that their self-denial behaviors do not lead to any improvement in the relationship and feel that they are exploited by their partners, they get very disappointed and exhausted. One possible primary reason behind women's surrendering behaviors is traditional gender roles in which a female partner is responsible for taking care of her husband and her children, and makes them her priorities in life. A male partner, on the other hand, is only bread-winner of his family. The Turkish Statistical Institute (TUIK) reported in March 2017 that the participation rate to labor force was 31.5% for women while it was 71.6% for men. The same institute stated that as the degree of education increased, women's participation rate in the labor force also rose up. It claimed that the participation rate in the labor force of illiterate women was 16.1%, of the ones having secondary education was 26.6.%, of high-school graduates was 32.7%, of undergraduates was 71.6%. It can be said that these numbers reflect the impact of gender roles on this issue.

Being a Good Parent and a Good Spouse Ensures a True Intimate Relationship between the Partners

When couples have a child, they change their priorities and shape their life routines according to their child's needs. Especially, couples display their gender roles regarding how well a mother and a father should be (Kayser & Himle, 1994). Thus, for the mothers, raising and protecting children, and providing feeding opportunities to them become critical tasks in their lives while for the fathers, playing with the children, providing sheltering facilities to them, and spending lots of money for their welfare are the major burdens on them. Based on these roles, they believe they have a satisfactory marriage life.

However, in reality, as I encounter in my counseling sessions, couples are suffocated into these parenting roles prescribed by the culture. For example, in Turkey, a woman (having a career or not), is expected to stay at home and nurture her children, and even not to return her career life due to the children. A man, on the other hand, is expected to provide adequate money and organize material facilities at home, and not to be included in his spouse's tasks like cooking, washing dishes, etc. In such a marriage, couples do their own tasks and do not help each other in both doing daily chores and taking care of the kids. Thus, women have more responsibilities than men. In this situation, couples usually forget their own psychological needs (e.g., spending a qualitative time with the spouse like a private dinner, a special holiday. etc.) and start to argue about how routine their life is and how emotionally distant they are when there are no children around them. Specifically, female partners complain about how insensitive their partners are while male partners grumble about the fact that their partners do not pay attention to their physical and psychological satisfaction like sex life as they prioritize their children in their existence.

Behaving according to the Romantic Ideals Leads to Endless Love between Partners

As you see in your counseling occasions, partners believe that each one should behave in accordance with the romantic ideals or standards depicted by television films, movies, or romantic comedies. Especially, they think that the romantic companionship, for example, is based on love at first sight and if such an event does not occur in one of the partners, the relationship does not last long. To

Baucom and Epstein (1990), the major challenge in romantic relations is that couples have wishful thinking shaped by one's romantic desires in which the relational facts are not consciously or unconsciously taken into consideration. These imaginary romantic life beliefs lead them to form the criteria for excellent romantic relationships. If one of the partners cannot fulfill those criteria, he or she is not the one and the relationship should be terminated.

To cultivation theory, mass media channels have a great impact on creating a prevalent notion about ideal romantic partnership via reality shows, marriage programs, movies etc. (Gerbner & Gross, 1976). Whether the information dispersed is true or not, repeated exposure to them causes many couples to have illusionary assumptions regarding how romanticism should be maintained and how a perfect marriage should be attained (Eggermont, 2004; Galician, 2004; Signorelli, 1991). They think that these assumptions are reachable entities if a couple behaves relying on them.

Based on Galician (2004, p. 55)'s myths of love, I try to illustrate the common problems Turkish couples have due to their romantic ideals.

"To attract and keep a man, a woman should look like a model or a centerfold"

In counseling sessions, it is possible to see a female client complaining about her weight, height, etc. – in her physical appearance – and seeing it as a reason behind the conflicts with her partner. Female clients usually believe that if they are very beautiful naturally or with aesthetic interventions, their partner's love will be endless. Therefore, there are many females dissatisfied with their true selves. Such a discontent leads to negative interactions between couples. It results in a materialistic love rather than unconditional love between the companions.

"The man should not be shorter, weaker, younger, poorer, or less successful than the woman"

In Turkey, female partners usually believe that if a man is very rich and has high social status in the society, and looks very well physically, he can protect his romantic partner efficiently and provide sufficient resources for his companion as well as his children. This idea is pertinent to the collectivistic cultures in which patriarchal units are more dominant than matriarchal units in the society. Man is regarded as breadwinner while woman is considered as mother and landlady at home.

"The love of a good and faithful true woman can change a man from a 'beast' into a 'prince'"

I encounter many female clients who say that "I believed I could change his faulty behaviors, bad habits with my profound love, but I couldn't. Why? Am I insufficient to him?" Especially, female clients think that formal union like engagement, marriage, etc. can alter their male partners' behaviors and thoughts which they find as harmful, bad, disgusting, and so on. However, in reality, such an understanding is not possible. Male partners usually struggle with the control-freak partners who try to organize them in the way they would like to do so. In this relationship, male partners are under the surveillance of their female partners and there is no private room to hide from them. Thus, over time, male partners escape from this situation via long business visits, love affairs, and so on. In a counseling session where a couple has such a relationship, female and male partners would usually like to terminate their relationship as they think it is not satisfactory in emotional and psychological terms.

"Bickering and fighting a lot mean that a man and a woman really love each other passionately"

I see in counseling that the couples who believe this idea think "hatred is related to love." At the beginning of their relationship, they consider that these fights are the signs of extreme attention of each partner and hence they are seen as a normal communication. However, over time, they understand that their companionship hangs on by a thread. This is why their relationship is very fragile and fluctuating in accordance with psychologically hurtful arguments. The lack of complementarity in the relationship leads to many disharmonies among couples.

"In real life, actors and actresses are often very much like the romantic characters they portray"

As couples are exposed to many romantic comedies, movies, or films in the mass media, they begin to think that the actors and actresses who are couples live in the way they depicted in these social materials. In counseling sessions, I have a couple who say that "We want to live a romantic life illustrated in Turkish movie called Magnificent Century in which Suleiman the Magnificent" – one of the most successful Ottoman Sultans and Hurrem Sultan (Aleksandra Lisowska) – one of the women from his harem who could manage to become an official wife of the sultan for the first time in the Ottoman history. Since the couples never acquire this kind of romantic relationship, they feel high levels of displeasure and grievance.

Culture and Traditional Gender Roles

In addition to dysfunctional relationship beliefs, culture has a great impact on how romantic love is perceived and experienced (Dion & Dion, 1993; 1996; Goode, 1959; Levine, Sato, Hashimoto, & Verma, 1995). There are cultural differences in comprehending how a romantic affair should be. For collectivistic cultures where the welfare of the others in the society is more pivotal than one's own well-being (Hofstede, 1984), the kinships and extended family bonds are essential determinants in choosing a potential romantic partner (Lamanna & Riedmann, 2009). The possible partner should be suitable to the norms and standards of extended family and should acquire the family's approval. On the other hand, for individualistic cultures where self-actualization and achievement of individual purposes in his life is more significant than societal goals (Hofstede, 1984), romantic love represents the act of going after one's individual desires and provides the opportunity to accomplish one's self-exploration and self-determination (Lamanna & Riedmann, 2009). In these cultures, marriage is based on romantic love rather than arranged interviews made by the families.

Turkey, one of the developing countries in the world, can be considered as collectivistic, conventional, and patriarchal society where the cultural norms emphasizing the collectivistic principles such as interdependence, loyalty to family values, societal benefits, social status, men's decisive roles in each area of life and so on are salient in interpersonal relationships (Hortaçsu, 2007; Kağıtçıbaşı, 2005). Despite an increase in Western type of love and marriages in city lives, there are still arranged marriages in Turkey (Atalay, Kontas, Beyazit, & Madenoglu, 1992). Therefore, togetherness between the families of the partners and between themselves is very critical for healthy companionships.

In Turkey, families can display enormous versatility in accordance with their social status, educational history and degree of religious tendency (Delevi & Bugay, 2010). Families where parents have high degrees of education or/and have middle / high socioeconomic status, or/and have secular opinions regarding family life encourage their youth to have a romantic relationship they would like to be part in and marry the one they love. They insist on letting their youth make his or her decision about potential romantic companions. On the other hand, families where parents have low degrees of education or/and or/and have low socioeconomic status, or/and have conservative ideas about family life do not allow their youth to have a romantic partnership in which they do not approve. Although those families let their youth experience romantic relations, they would still like to intervene the youth's last decision about the partner whether he or she is suitable to his or her family's norms. In both urban and rural areas of Turkey, the parent who holds the economic resources of the family – usually the fathers – is the decision-maker in this process.

Moreover, the impact of family structures on romantic affairs also includes the influence of traditional gender roles on these relations, which are shaped by the family patterns one grew up with. Gender roles can be defined as the cultural standards for how to be feminine or masculine in society (O'Neil, 1981). Traditional gender roles are the thinking patterns pertinent to how a family unit should be constructed and how work in the family should be disseminated in reference to one's gender. Based on these roles, men are expected to gain money and provide economic help to his family, while women are expected to devote themselves to their children by nurturing and caring for them (Basow & Johnson, 2000; Eagly, Wood, & Diekman, 2000).

To Sakallı and Curun (2001), Turkish males and females who embrace traditional gender roles comply with the common societal rules depicted in Turkish culture. In their study, they found Turkish females believe that men should adopt self-assured and decisive roles in romantic companionships. Turkish males, on the other hand, believe that women should obey the rules they form in romantic bonds. Thus, Turkish males attempt to control their partners' physical appearance as well as psychological stance in their lives. Especially, Turkish males intervene in their romantic partners' private preferences such as the places they would like to go, the dresses they want to wear, the career goals they would like to achieve, etc. In such a relationship, women are expected to fulfill their responsibilities to the romantic relationship by behaving according to the standards men create.

When analyzing problematic and dysfunctional relationship beliefs in a couple client, it is helpful to take into account both individual and cultural factors. As these cognitive errors are formed through social experiences, family patterns and gender roles become two important components determining whether a couple will have a healthy or unhealthy relationship, whether they will have a happy ending, and whether they will maintain their harmonious dance between themselves.

Intervention Strategies

In this section, I try to briefly summarize culturally sensitive approaches for ameliorating cognitive distortions in Turkish couples.

Pinpoint the Goals of Each Partner in Order to Understand their Motivation to Alter their Romantic Lives

In Turkey, you recognize that it is women who usually initiate the idea for a couple to seek family counseling as they see themselves as being responsible for saving their family life due to their traditional gender roles depicted by a proverb called "Nesters are female birds – Yuvayı disi kuş yapar." In this regard, you should ask questions like "Who made the idea that we should go to a couple counseling?" In this way, you can understand which partner is more committed to the counseling process, leading to a change in their romantic relationship.

Identify the Dysfunctional Family of Origin Rules in Each Partner

It is the most important technique in couple counseling in Turkey. As family rules are very significant in Turkish culture, you should examine parents' relationship quality and communication patterns with each partner. As I see in my counseling sessions, couples usually adopt their parents' maladaptive conflict resolution strategies which are based on dysfunctional relationship beliefs like "Any argument in relationship leads to its termination" or "Being very intimate in a romantic relationship makes the one vulnerable to his or her partner" by modeling their parents' behaviors since their childhood. To identify these beliefs, you can use such questions as "How did your parents get on with each other? What did they call each other?, etc."

Besides this, you should also take into account past relationship experiences starting from late adolescence by asking questions like "Which romantic relationship lasted longer in your past?", "How did your relationships end? And why?", "Which song did you prefer when you experienced the first break-up?, etc." Especially, the question related to the songs is very effective for understanding the clients' perspectives toward break-ups. Turkish couples usually prefer to listen to songs which include the words indicating lots of pain like arabesque music. The clients who very frequently listen to such songs perceive the situation as a deadly end. They feel very intense sorrow, leading them even to commit suicide, or a crime like killing the one who wants to break up from him or her.

Use Assignments to Increase Couples' Awareness

Keeping a diary or writing letters to each other are very effective for Turkish couples who want to understand each other's feelings and thoughts accurately.

Use Enactment Technique to Figure out the Problematic Areas of Couples' Relationships

In Turkey, you can use such topics as the use of social media (arguing about giving password to the partner or not), the social activities couples are included together like their friends' weddings, football matches, the shopping mall adventures, family reunions in feasts, holiday experiences, etc. to see their communication patterns. Especially, family reunions in feasts give important cues about how couples consider each other's behaviors. For example, a wife wants to go to a holiday with her husband while he wants to visit his parents during the Ramadan feast when all business sectors are closed. This situation creates lots of arguments among Turkish couples. If you give this topic in your counseling, you will understand different expectations of each partner regarding to the holiday time.

Help Couple Clients Produce Alternative Ways of Thinking and Behaving in their Conflictual Situations

To achieve this aim, you should ask questions like "Based on your family of origin experiences or the occurrences in your present romantic relationship, what evidence assists your opinion? What can be an alternative comment for your partner's behavior?" In Turkey, couples who have communication problems embrace their families' ideas about their situation without questioning. For example, a man who is raised in a very conventional family expects all caring issues from his wife and any lack of fulfilling that responsibility is a sign of a lack of love for him. When he tells his mother his idea, she can interpret the situation in the same way. Thus, he gets confirmation by his mother and responds to his wife accordingly. Thus, teaching couples alternative thinking pathways is an important tool for developing their romantic relationships.

Case Example

Aslı, age 35, is a human resources manager who has been working in that area for 13 years. Three years ago she married Kaya, age 32, a veterinary in a special clinic, working in that place for seven years. They have one daughter – Zeynep – 2 years old. Aslı wants to advance in her career and become a manager assistant of her CEO in her company. Yet, Kaya wants her to pay more attention to their marriage and family life. They conflict a lot about this issue and feel that something goes wrong between them. In this case, firstly, I try to find out dysfunctional family of origin rules in each partner by asking what kind of family they were raised in (conventional, modern, or very conservative, etc.). Especially, I want them to identify what are the expectations they have from a marriage (from the opposite sex partner). Based on their expectations, I comprehend how they look at traditional gender roles, and family life. I encourage the couple to openly discuss their ideas and thoughts about their relationship in order to make their dysfunctional beliefs clear. After the discussion, effective communication and problem-solving skills are emphasized so as to help them have the feelings of acceptance and commitment in their relationship.

Conclusions and Recommendations

I try to briefly summarize the potential pitfalls we should avoid when counseling Turkish couples.

Do Not Have Any Ethnocentric Thoughts or Feelings in Counseling

As Turkish couples represent a different cultural world to you, you should avoid thinking that your own culture is an exceptional one. If any feeling related to this idea occurs, your counselees will contemplate that you make an unfavorable cultural comparison and overlook them rather than focus on their problems.

Do Not Evaluate the State of Your Counselees Based on a Stereotypical Understanding

As a counselor, you should try to get to know the values of Turkish culture in an open-minded way. You should avoid considering Turkish people as barbarian, or narrow-minded about religion.

Do Not Overstate Individual-based Counseling as the Counselees Come from a Collectivistic Culture

In counseling, when using necessary intervention techniques for the Turkish couples, we should consider them as the ones who are the part of their families. Despite all family members' not participating into the counseling session, we should look at the couples in a holistic way (in the family environment they are raised)

References

Atalay, B., Kontas, M., Beyazit, S., & Madenoglu, K. (1992). *Investigation of Turkish family structure*. Ankara: State Planning Organization.

Baldwin, M. W. (1992). Relational schemas and the processing of social information. Psychological Bulletin, 112(3), 461–484.

Basow, S. A., & Johnson, K. (2000). Predictors of homophobia in female college students. Sex Roles, 42, 391–404.

Baucom, D. H., Epstein, N., Sayers, S., & Sher, T. S. (1989). The role of cognitions in marital relationships: Definitional, methodological and conceptual issues. Journal of Counseling Clinical Journal, 57, 31–38.

Baucom, D. H., & Epstein, N. (1990). *Cognitive-behavioral marital therapy*. New York: Brunner/Mazel.

Beck, A. T. (1963). Thinking and depression I: Idiosyncratic content and cognitive distortions. Archives of General Psychiatry, 9, 324–333.

Chen, S. (2001). The role of theories in mental representation and their use in social perception: A theory-based approach to significant-other representations and transference. In G. B. Moskowitz (Ed.), *Cognitive social psychology: The Princeton symposium on the legacy and future of social cognition* (pp. 125–142). Mahwah, NJ: Erlbaum.

Dattilio, F. M. (2010). *Cognitive-behavioral therapy with couples and families: A comprehensive guide for clinicians*. New York: The Guilford Press.

Delevi, R., & Bugay, A. (2010). Understanding change in romantic relationship expectations of international female students from Turkey. Contemporary Family Therapy, 32, 257–272.

Dion, K. K., & Dion, K. L. (1993). Individualistic and collectivistic perspectives on gender and the cultural context of love and intimacy. Journal of Social Issues, 49(3), 53–69.

Dion, K. K., & Dion, K. L. (1996). Cultural perspectives on romantic love. Personal Relationships, 3, 5–17.

Eagly, A. H., Wood, W., & Diekman, A. B. (2000). Social role theory of sex differences and similarities: A current appraisal. In T. Eckes & H. M. Trautner (Eds.), *The developmental social psychology of gender* (pp. 123–174). Mahwah, NJ: Lawrence Erlbaum Associates.

Eggermont, S. (2004). Television viewing, perceived similarity, and adolescents' expectations of a romantic partner. *Journal of Broadcasting and Electronic Media*, 48(2), 244–265.

Epstein, N., & Eidelson, R. J. (1981). Unrealistic beliefs of clinical couples: Their relationship to expectations, goals and satisfaction. *American Journal of Family Therapy*, 9, 13–22.

Filipovic, S., Vukosavljevic-Gvozden, T., & Opacic, G. (2016). Irrational beliefs, dysfunctional emotions, and marital adjustment: A structural model. *Journal of Family Issues*, 37 (16), 2333–2350.

Fincham, F. D., & Bradbury, T. N. (1989). The impact of attributions in marriage: An individual difference analysis. *Journal of Social and Personal Relationships*, 6, 69–85.

Fiske, A. P., & Haslam, N. (1996). Social cognition is thinking about relationships. *Current Directions in Psychological Science*, 5, 143–148.

Galician, M. L. (2004). *Sex, love, and romance in the mass media: Analysis and criticism of unrealistic portrayals and their influence*. Mahwah, NJ: Lawrence Erlbaum.

Gerbner, G., & Gross, L. (1976). Living with television: The violence profile. *Journal of Communication*, 26(2), 172–199.

Gizir, C. A. (2013). An investigation of the relationship beliefs of the university students regarding gender and dating status. *Education and Science*, 38(170), 372–383.

Goode, W. J. (1959). The theoretical importance of love. *American Sociological Review*, 24, 38–47.

Hamamcı, Z. (2005). Dysfunctional relationship beliefs in marital conflict. *Journal of Rational-Emotive & Cognitive-Behavior Therapy*, 23(3), 245–261.

Hofstede, G. (1984). *Culture's consequences: International differences in work-related values*. Thousand Oaks, CA: Sage Publications.

Holmes, B. M. (2004). Romantic partner ideals and dysfunctional relationship beliefs cultivated through popular media messages: Implications for relationship satisfaction. (Unpublished Doctorate Dissertation). University of Massachusetts, Amherst, USA.

Horney, K. (1937). *The neurotic personality of our time*. New York: W. W. Norton & Company.

Horney, K. (1945). *Our inner conflicts*. New York: W. W. Norton & Company.

Hortacsu, N. (2003). Marriage in Turkey. In R. R. Hamon & B. B. Ingoldsby (Eds.), *Mate selection across cultures*. Thousand Oaks, CA: Sage.

Jowett, B., & Pelliccia, H. (1996). *Symposium: The Benjamin Jowett translation*. New York: Modern Library.

Kağıtçıbaşı, Ç. (2005). Autonomy and relatedness in cultural context: Implications for self and family. *Journal of Cross-Cultural Psychology*, 36(4), 403–422.

Kayser, K., & Himle, D. P. (1994). Dysfunctional beliefs about intimacy. *Journal of Cognitive Psychotherapy: An International Quarterly*, 8(2), 127–140.

Kelly, G. A. (1955). *The psychology of personal constructs*. New York: W. W. Norton & Company.

Knee, C. R. (1998). Implicit theories of relationships: Assessment and prediction of romantic relationship initiation, coping and longevity. *Journal of Personality and Social Psychology*, 74(2), 360–370.

Kurdek, L. A. (1993). Predicting marital dissolution: A 5-year prospective longitudinal study of newlywed couples. *Journal of Personality and Social Psychology*, 64, 221–242.

Lamanna, M. A., & Riedmann, A. (2009). *Marriages and families: Making choices in a diverse society*. Belmont, CA: Wadsworth.

Levine, R., Sato, S., Hashimoto, T., & Verma, J. (1995). Love and marriage in eleven cultures. *Journal of Cross-Cultural Psychology*, 26(5), 554–571.
O'Neil, J. M. (1981). Patterns of gender role conflict and strain: Sexism and fear of femininity in men's lives. *Personnel & Guidance Journal*, 60, 203–210.
Polster, E., & Polster, M. (1973). *Gestalt therapy integrated: Contours of theory and practice*. New York: Brunner/Mazel.
Regan, P. (2011). *Close relationships*. Abingdon: Routledge.
Sakallı, N., & Curun, F. (2001). Romantik ilişkilerle ilgili kalıpyargılara karşı tutumlar. *Türk Psikiyatri Dizini*, 22, 31–45.
Signorelli, N. (1991). Adolescents and ambivalence toward marriage: A cultivation analysis. *Youth and Society*, 19, 121–149.
Thibaut, J. W., & Kelley, H. H. (1959). *The social psychology of groups*. New York: Wiley & Sons.
Young, J. E., Klosko, S., & Weishaar, M. E. (2003). *Schema therapy: A practitioner's guide*. New York: Guilford Press.

Additional Resources

Dwairy, M., & El-Jamil, F. (2016). Counseling Arab and Muslim clients. In P. B. Pedersen, W. J. Lonner, J. G. Draguns, J. E. Trimble, & M. R. Scharraon-del Rio (Eds.), *Counseling across cultures* (pp. 185–204). Los Angeles, CA: Sage.
Hortaçsu, N. (2007). Family-versus couple-initiated marriages in Turkey: Similarities and differences over the family life cycle. *Asian Journal of Applied Psychology*, 10, 103–116.
Kağıtçıbaşı, Ç. (2007). *Family, self and human development across cultures: Theory and applications* (2nd ed.). Mahwah, NJ: Erlbaum.
Poyrazlı, Ş., Doğan, S., & Eskin, M. (2013). Counseling and psychotherapy in Turkey: Western theories and culturally inclusive methods. In R. Moodley, U. Gielen, & R. Wu (Eds.), *Handbook of counseling and psychotherapy in an international context* (pp. 404–414). New York: Routledge.
Selin, H. (2014). *Parenting across cultures: Childrearing, motherhood and fatherhood in non-Western cultures*. New York: Springer.

7

STRESSORS UPON MARRIAGE IN THE BARTER ECONOMY OF CUBA

Miriam Moreno-Duany

Introduction

For years Cuba was closed to the American people due to the embargo of 1961 placed on Cuba after Castro's changes within the island. (Department of State, 2019) As a result of the separation between these two countries, curiosity about the island began to develop with the passing of the years. In 1959, a young and handsome "Robin Hood" (Perrottet, 2019, p. 3) took power, by force, promising its people to take money from the rich and give it to the poor. That "hero" who responds to the name of Fidel Castro, as is supposed to be, had overwhelming support, even from rich people. Probably 90% of Cubans adored him, for several reasons. The youth looked up to him as a role model, a brave lawyer with the gift of the word. The older generations saw him as the person who was going to end all the corruption, crime, and injustice that existed at that time. Women loved him for his beauty, his physical strength and his exquisite verbiage. He was able to stand before a crowd of hardworking men and women and speak for eight hours at a time. He made promises to the people dreaming of a better future that Cubans still await. However, at that time everyone had at least one reason to support him: everyone wanted the injustices to come to an end, and so far, 59 years later, the children, grandchildren, and great-grandchildren of that generation continue to hope for a better life.

Cuba has kept secret how its people really live. It was closed off to the world for more than 15 years and now many speculate what is the true way of life for Cubans. Most of Cuban society is completely controlled by the government. The government censures anything that contradicts government policy as disseminated by the Cuban government around the world. Many speculate and wonder how Cubans live; everything that comes from Cuba is a sensation amongst different populations in the USA. However, the reality for the Cuban people is far from what the propaganda that Fidel Castro spent years broadcasting to the world. Cuba has been under the revolution for almost 60 years, with Fidel Castro at the head of the island. In 2006, his brother Raúl Castro replaced him temporarily due to illness and in 2008 he formally replaced him as president of the Council of State and Ministers. Raúl Castro was in charge for about 10 years until June 2018, when he appointed a new president, Miguel Díaz-Canel. He follows the same type of government, regulations and responds to the Castro's family interests (Faiola, 2018).

The island country of Cuba stands in the middle of the Caribbean Sea, shaped as an alligator, with a population of 11,433,588 people (World Bank, 2018). Cuba has existed under different types of political systems, including democratic mandate, dictatorship, and socialism. Before Castro gained political power, Cuba was a dictatorship but with open relations with United States and other countries. In an article written to the Smithsonian, Historian Louis Perez stated that "Havana was then what Las Vegas has become" (Geiling, 2007). Americans could access Havana to gamble, drink, dance, and have adventures. Famous actors, singers, and dancers, such as Frank Sinatra, Rita Hayworth, Carl Gable, Errol Flynn, Montgomery Clift, and many others would visit the island and enjoy the weather, the casinos, and the Cuban culture. Under Batista's regime, Cuba was the center for organized crime for the United States, and officials in Cuba protected this. In 1957, casinos were a major industry reaching earnings of up to $500,000. It is estimated that there were about 270 brothels, and about 11,500 women were part of the prostitution scene (Perez, 2006).

Even the famous American journalist, novelist, and short story writer Ernest Hemingway spent long periods of his life in Cuba; his residence was Finca Vigia from 1939 until 1960 (Ferrero, 2008), ("Lookout Farm") intermittently during the last two decades of his life. The estate was dear to his heart. He owned a house on the island, and that house witnessed the birth of at least eight literary works including *The Old Man and the Sea* for which he received the Pulitzer Prize for Fiction in 1953. Finca Vigia is located 16 kilometers east of Havana and is currently a museum. Visitors are forbidden inside the house for fear of damaging of the writer's personal belongings (Herlihy-Mera, 2017, p. 37). Due to the fact that Hemingway was a fan of fishing, he created "The Ernest Hemingway International Bill fishing Tournament" which continues to be held in Cuba and is considered one of the oldest fishing tournaments in the world. That is the reason why on the island there is currently a tourist place that is presented today as the famous "Hemingway Marina" located on Avenida 248 y 5A, Santa Fe, Havana, Cuba, with access to all those who can pay the price (Marina Hemingway Cuba, 2015).

Cuba is known for its music, its rich Afro-Cuban culture, food, and rich culture. However, tourists are often exposed to the beautiful settings that are created for them by the government. They can only see the marvelous colors of the old cars, the colorful typical clothes and hats, the smiles Cubans show to the visitors, but tourists are not aware of the daily struggles to provide for the family, to find food to put on the table, the hardship of finding a suitable home – all of these struggles are left behind curtains. The happiness that lives innate within the Cuban people is what is shown to the tourists that come visit the island. Due to the fact that the miseries of the Cuban people are not spoken off, Cubans have found a way to make a comfortable living using the tourism that is rampant all year round. Follow along to unveil the Cuban reality.

It is important for the reader to know that Cuba has many underworlds that are not allowed to be openly discussed. The author of this chapter was born and raised in Cuba, while she came at a young age to the United States, she keeps close contact with family that still reside on the island. Having close contact with these individuals makes this information a possibility to be written and shared with the outside world. As previously mentioned, Cuba has been under many different presidents, but under Castro's mandate many changes came about on the island. These changes included family relations, the woman's role, child upbringing, education, medicine, and marriage. For this particular chapter the change in marriage and its evolution throughout the many years of the revolution will be discussed.

Family Structure in Cuba

In Cuba, it is customary for men to marry or to live with just one woman. Usually, the lower the educational status, the more children people have. Individuals with a higher educational level tend to have one or two children. Abortions are common and not prohibited by law; to a certain extent abortion is expected if the child was not planned or if the child will have some sort of congenital malformation that can be previously diagnosed during gestation. In this day and age, men have children with different women. Marriage is barely seen, and consensual relationships are more common. Children are always expected to be raised and be at home with the mother. The woman is the "pillar" of the home, and she is designated to raise the children, maintain the home with the cleaning, cooking, laundry, and work outside of the home.

Due to the lack of housing that is part of the daily struggle, it is common for three generations to live under the same roof. For example, if the grandparents have a child, when that child marries the husband comes into the household, and when they have a child that marries, the man or the wife would come to live under the same house. This constitutes three generations living in the same household.

Family and Marriage before the Revolution

Cuba was colonized by the Spaniards, so reasonably many of the customs that dictated Cuban culture came from them. The Spaniards had very old-fashioned traditions that were adapted into Cuban culture: "[t]he ideals of chivalry dictated conduct, piety, honor, valor, courtesy, chastity and loyalty" (Skaine, 2004, p. 6). Historically, women were expected to stay home, raise the children and take care of the household. It was an established system within the household, and anything different from that was not easily accepted. Before 1959, when the revolution came, the main breadwinner was the male, and although the Spaniards passed on many of their traditions and way of life, Cuba decided to steer away from the matriarchal traditions upheld by the culture in Spain (Skaine, 2004).

It was common for the males living in the city to travel to the countryside looking for possible mates, if they liked the woman or "fell in love" they would mount them on their horse and take them back to the city. They would start a family and marriage was left on the sidelines. This was the case of Tania and Pablo; he lived in the Santiago de Cuba; he was traveling outside the city and landed in a small "pueblo" called Los Negros that consisted of about 20 houses. There was no electricity – it was in fact a foreign concept. Pablo saw Tania walking outside; she was only 14 years old. He pursued her and within a month's time he had taken her to the city to live. This was a commonality back in the 1930s and 1940s. They had six children. They were legally married in 1961, two years after the revolution; all of their children were born with the youngest being 6 years old. Having a "big family" was common practice, as family was an important part of the culture. Marriages would normally have more than three children, and for men to have children outside of the marriage was not criticized. Religion was an important part of the Cuban culture as well, with Catholicism being the major denomination. Taking this into consideration, there were many women who resided within the city limits that would be required to marry before entering a relationship with a man. Living out of wedlock was left for the prostitutes or the less affluent families. In Havana, there was the popular Chinatown, which still exists today, but back in the day it was famous for its brothels, as briefly mentioned above. Chinese people began immigrating to Cuba in 1847; due to work contract, they had to work in the sugar cane plantations. According to the historian Le Riverend (2007) around 1850 the sugar industry was improving, and the new technology was in need of more quality workers. In Cuba, slaves were obligated to work without a break for long hours. Cuba began to make massive contracts for Chinese as semi-slaves to operate the machinery. Later on, some of them escaped from different parts of China for political oppression and looking for a better life. Nowadays, Chinatown still exists but no Chinese individuals live there, and brothels are no longer part of the scene. (Vargas, 2017)

Family and Marriage after the Revolution

With the start of the revolution changes started happening in the island. Many believe that Cuba has stopped in time: "it is like a picture frozen in time," say many Cuban Americans. This image has been created in people's minds because there is no progress in the country. The economy is dead in its track, people do not have the means to put food on the table, much less to build or restore their homes. For many foreigners, Cuba is a place to have fun and to visit a time of the 1940s, 1950s, and 1960s; however for those that live in the reality of Cuba know of the oppression, the hypocrisy, and that immense poverty that lives within the country. During the 1960s the brigade "Patria o Muerte" was created by Fidel Castro to increment the literacy rate. This consisted of professionals (men and women) receiving paid leave and teaching in rural areas. This continued with the nationalization of enterprise and services to the community. By the end of the 1960s women became part of the production industry, "[w]omen who had previously never worked outside of the home travelled across the interior countryside as teachers, agricultural workers and administrators" (Perez, 2006, p. 282). As result, this brought changes within the household; women were now expected to work outside the home, clean the house, bear children and raise them as well as be of support to the husband.

Due to the hardship of the Cuban people, they have found creative ways to support the family. There are traditional marital roles, but it is common for "... [Cubans] to engage in black market activities ..." (Skaine, 2004, p. 17) due to the lack of incentives the government has to offer. According to the National Center for Statistics in 2016 the divorce rate at a total of 31,598, compared to 2015 which was at 33,174. This may be due to the fact that legal marriage is becoming less of a commonality and conjugal living is becoming more of the standard (Skaine, 2004). As a result of the island's meager living standards, it basically lives off the tourists that visit the island all year round. It is common for a taxi driver to make more than a doctor (Skaine, 2004), and for marriages or partners to convene a story where one of partners lives a double life. The story would go something like this: a poor single mother trying to make ends meet, abandoned by her child's father is seeking love, reasonably the "love" she finds would be in the arms of a tourist that can pay for her comfortable living. This would entail the man or the woman (most commonly the woman) having a relationship with a tourist while still having a formal relationship with a live-in partner. This would be of mutual agreement and it would not be frowned upon since it is a way to provide for the family and to have a better standard of living than most of the Cuban population. Infidelity runs rampant on both sides (either man or woman) due to the current economic structure that creates a lot of stress and forces people to live double lives out of necessity. The desperation has increased to astronomical levels that men allow their girlfriend or wife to date a tourist to provide for the family. The word *machismo* "... var[ies] from country to country, yet as a vestige of patriarchy machismo is a set of expectations for men where they assert dominance and superiority over women" (Fox & Zagumny, 2017, p. 98). While it is true that *machismo* is still part of the culture, the younger population are not preoccupied with fidelity, they are more concerned with having a comfortable living. While traditional marriage roles still exist for some, others are far from what traditional marital roles were at one point. The case example of Jose and Susy will help in understanding what the author is trying to convey.

Counseling in Cuban Culture

The terms counseling and/or counselor in Cuba are not a common one. The terms used are psychotherapy, psychologist, and psychiatrist. In Cuba, a medical degree takes six years to study for, and five years for all others. The psychiatrist works closely with psychologist, and they provide psychotherapy on a regular basis. Being a psychiatrist in Cuba is of high prestige, as well as a psychologist. In Cuba, there are no licensing boards; during your time of study you practice with patients in the community and a combination of theory and practice is utilized throughout all years of study. Even though there are no licensing boards, in order to graduate the student must take a national exam in order to validate the degree. It happens once a year for all provinces. In 2015, the American Psychological Association sent three psychologists to Cuba in search of the benefits of the healthcare system. They found that “American psychologists have much more to learn from Cuban psychologists, such as the nation’s integration of physical and mental health care, its emphasis on prevention and early intervention and its resourcefulness in the face of limited resources” (Clay, 2015). Through this exploration, the team of psychologists figured out that Cuba holds a more holistic approach and working as a team is of great value and expected within the system.

The term mental health counselor is not understood by the community, but at the end of the day counseling happens on a daily basis. In actuality, the theory that is most commonly used throughout the island is Cognitive Behavioral Therapy (CBT) and solution focused therapy is becoming more rampant. There are highly qualified psychologists and psychiatrist that specialize in couple counseling. However, older couples do not partake in therapy due to the taboo of going in search of a therapist since it was highly stigmatized as part of the culture. In this group of individuals, it is a belief that family problems are personal and should be kept within the confines of the family. Nevertheless, younger couples are more open to dialogue and search for help and for this reason they are more prone to seek out a therapist to help them. Given the high *machismo* that resides in the country there are those professionals (psychologists) that lack the ability to partialize themselves with one of the spouses. The story of Maria and Alberto is a perfect example to showcase this comment. Maria and Alberto decided to seek help since their marriage had been struggling. When they sit in front of the psychologist, Maria tells her part of the story and quickly Alberto interrupts and starts telling his part turning things to his favor. By the end of his story, the psychologist starts responding from a male perspective, blaming everything on Maria. The result of the session was the Maria ended up crying, they left the session and never went back. Many years passed and while they are still together, they never went back to therapy. This is an example of a psychologist that allowed his *machismo* to take over the session. While this is not common it can happen, as shown with this case. However, this was about 35 years ago, and the problems that existed in Cuba 35 years ago are not the ones that exist today. Although couple counseling is available in Cuba, it is not widely utilized as a priority for families struggling with basic needs. There is also the belief that a therapist will not solve their problems, and therefore they do not take the time to ask for their help.

Case Study

Jose and Susy live within the island. Jose is a 40-year-old male and Susy is 35. They have a 5-year-old daughter in common and they reside in the province of Santiago de Cuba. Jose and Susy have been together, living under the same roof for about ten years; they lived apart the first six months, but due to the housing conditions in Cuba partners quickly start cohabiting. Jose's grandparents gave him a small piece of the garage where he could build a home for his family. He works as a bartender; his pay does not surpass the $10 CUC mark a month. He works in a bar that uses Cuban pesos, making less than he needs to provide for himself and his family. Susy does not work because she does not have a marketable educational level that can obtain her a decent paying job. They do not have family nearby that can support them on a daily basis by taking care of their daughter. Jose's mother lives close, but she is taking care of Jose's grandmother whom is old and senile. To work with the tourism industry there are requirements such as speaking basic English and taking the courses required through the Tourism Ministry, although, it is known that with a "connection" or a "good recommendation" it is easier to obtain a job in this particular industry. It is not an easy task, and it leaves people hopeless of obtaining a position with the tourism industry.

However, given the number of tourists that visit the country on a yearly basis from all over the world (Spain, France, England, Ecuador, Mexico, etc.) it is convenient and to a certain extent easier to reach a tourist by sleeping with them. This is the case with Susy. She and Jose devised a plan to "catch" an Ecuadoran who visits that island on different occasions throughout the year. Susy met him in a bar and started flirting with him. She quickly told him that she had a 5-year-old daughter, but that her husband had left her, and she was struggling making ends meet. He believed her story and after two or three visits they started a formal relationship. The man visits Cuba more regularly now since he goes to visit Susy. They always stay in hotels around the province of Santiago with the excuse that she cannot leave the province because of her daughter. When she goes to visit the man, Susy leaves her daughter with her dad in their home. There are times where she takes her, if the Ecuadoran wants to see the little girl, but their meetings are usually far away from the home. There have been other times where they have used Jose's mother's house as a meeting place. The man goes to visit

Susy and the child in this house, and while the grandmother is aware of the situation, she stays quiet and does not get involved in her son's decisions.

It is always appropriate to build rapport by getting to know the couple, each person on an individual case, and understand their need of their partner and of the relationship. Given that the main theoretical orientation used in the island is CBT, it would be appropriate to do some brief psychoeducation with the clients in order to help them understand the theory. It would also be important to talk about feelings and positive communication styles to be utilized when the spouses are speaking to each other. Even though CBT and Solution Focused Brief Therapy are the most commonly used theoretical orientation, it may be of benefit to implement Unconditional Positive Regard. According to Murphy (2015)

> When a person is acting in accord with their organismic valuing, valuing each self-experience as equally acceptable to all other self-experiences, they have low conditions of worth. When a person experiences high unconditional positive self-regard, behavior will be directed towards the satisfaction of needs that are more consistent with internal values and intrinsic aspirations. This means they will be less inclined to act in accord with conditions of worth. (p. 206)

It may be that the person's need to provide will lead them to act in deplorable and immoral things, such as living a double life. However, going off Murphy's statement it may be that both spouses' self-worth is low since one is committing the act, and the other is accepting and supporting it. It can be perceived that Jose is seeing his wife as merchandise to solve his daily struggles, and his wife is allowing and developing in this role. This goes beyond the spiritual beliefs that united them at one point in time.

There may be a use for career counseling, and helping the clients find more appropriate avenues for work. Maybe help Jose discuss his options in the tourism industry to work as a bartender. Also, find out Susy's background and/or abilities to help her apply for jobs that deal with tourists. There may be other job offers that are in Cuban pesos that could provide a better living, but the aspiration is always to work in the tourism industry. It may be of benefit to help Susy find resources within the community, this will help empower her and guide her to find other options for her life and the life of her family. Likewise, help Jose find the right courses to fulfill the requirements to bartend within the tourism industry. He could also find other bartender jobs that are better paying, not necessarily with tourism.

Conclusions and Recommendations

This chapter conveys the various family and clinical experiences of the author, as well as cited research. Cuba is complex social and political culture that in enigmatic to many. This chapter pays homage to Cuba traditions transmitted over many generations, known as "transicion de informacion de generacion a generacion."

References

Clay, R.A. (2015). Getting to know Cuba. *Monitor on Psychology*, 46(6), 30. www.apa.org/monitor/2015/06/cover-cuba.aspx.

Department of State. (n.d). A guide to the United States' history of recognition, diplomatic, and consular relations, by country since 1776: Cuba. Retrieved February 11, 2019, from https://history.state.gov/countries/cuba.

Estad O.N. (2006). Oficina Nacional de Estadistica. Retrieved October 29, 2018, from www.one.cu/.

Faiola, A. (2018, April 19). Castro rule in Cuba ends as Miguel Diaz-Canel confirmed in leadership change. *The Washington Post*. Retrieved February 3, 2019, from www.washingtonpost.com/world/the_americas/in-cubas-national-assembly-raul-castro-marks-last-moments-of-his-familys-rule/2018/04/18/82f82cd4-4293-11e8-b2dc-b0a403e4720a_story.html?noredirect=on&utm_term=.9af601532bc7.

Ferrero, G. R. (2008). Museo Finca Vigia celebrates its 45th birthday (1). *The Hemingway Review*, 2, 16. Retrieved from http://ezproxy.fau.edu/login?url=http://search.ebscohost.com/login.aspx?direct=true&AuthType=ip,cookie,url,uid&db=edsglr&AN=edsgcl.182525095&site=eds-live&scope=site.

Fox, B. L., & Zagumny, L. (2017). Organizational approaches to addressing machismo and sexuality in Cuba. *Journal of Ethnographic & Qualitative Research*, 12(2), 97–109.

Geiling, N. (2007, July 31). Before the revolution socialites and celebrities flocked to Cuba in the 1950s. *Smithsonian Magazine*. Retrieved February 3, 2019, from www.smithsonianmag.com/history/before-the-revolution-159682020/.

Herlihy-Mera, J. (2017). Cuba in Hemingway. The Hemingway Review, 36(2). https://doi.org/10.1353/hem/2017.0001.

Marina Hemingway Cuba: The largest marina in Cuba. (2015). Retrieved February 11, 2019, from www.hemingwaycuba.com/marina-hemingway-cuba.html.

Murphy, D., Demetriou, E., & Joseph, S. (2015). A cross sectional study to explore the mediating effect of intrinsic aspiration on the association between unconditional positive self-regard and posttraumatic growth. *Person-Centered & Experiential Psychotherapies*, 14 (3), 201.

Perez, L. A. (2006). *Cuba: Between reform and revolution* (3rd ed.). New York: Oxford University Press.

Perrottet, T. (2019). *Cuba Libre!: Che, Fidel, and the improbable revolution that changed world history*. New York: Random House.

Riverend, J. L. (2007). *Breve historia de Cuba*. La Habana: Editorial de Ciencias Sociales.

Skaine, R. (2004). *The Cuban family: Custom and change in an era of hardship*. Jefferson, NC: McFarland.

The World Bank. (2018). Population, total. Retrieved October 28, 2018, from https://data.worldbank.org/indicator/SP.POP.TOTL?locations=CU.

Vargas, Y. (2017, July 12). In Cuba, a Chinatown with no Chinese. *The Diplomat*. Retrieved February 3, 2019, from https://thediplomat.com/2017/07/in-cuba-a-chinatown-with-no-chinese/.

Additional Resources

www.ernesthemingwaycollection.com/about-hemingway/ernest-hemingway-in-cuba.
www.bbc.com/news/world-latin-america-19576144.
https://nypost.com/2016/11/27/inside-fidel-castros-life-of-luxury-and-ladies-while-country-starved/.
www.forbes.com/sites/billfrist/2015/06/08/cubas-most-valuable-export-its-healthcare-expertise/#6c7d9a15195e.

8

ADDRESSING DOMESTIC VIOLENCE WITH RUSSIAN COUPLES

Alena Prikhidko

Introduction

Domestic violence (DV), intimate partner violence (IPV), and discrimination against women are among the most pressing problems confronting Russia today (Horne, 1999; Hawkins, & Knox, 2014). For a long time, DV was considered a private matter in Russian society (Jäppinen, 2010), which was seen as a "dirty laundry not to be washed in public." According to World Gallup Poll in 1990s DV was considered by the majority of respondents as a private matter in which bystanders should not intervene, described by a saying "love birds argue having fun." However, at the end of the first decade of the 21st century Russian society started to understand the consequences of DV and the need to take an action (Prava zenshin – prava cheloveka, 2009).

However, traditional cultural norms of Russian gender culture dictate a dependent status for women (Horne, 1999). Thus, battered women are still concerned that should they leave the abuser, they will be unable to support themselves and their children. Moreover, the Russian proverb "he beats you, which means he loves you" shows that violent actions of male traditionally may be perceived as signs of care.

Additionally, sexual violence against women in Russia is widespread, and for many years this topic remained taboo. However, recently researchers and family counselors acknowledged the necessity of examining the effects of sex, age, and traditional values on Russian adults' perceptions of a sexual assault scenario (Diakonova-Curtis & Porter, 2014). Overall, Russian adults endorse more traditional roles for women than research indicates for adults in the USA, with men holding more traditional beliefs than women. When a man was given more authority and power, he was seen as more justified and was more likely to be exonerated when he committed a violent act against a woman (Diakonova-Curtis & Porter, 2014).

Marriage and family therapy (MFT) intensively develops in Russian society, however, there is no standardized counseling assistance for the family and this type of care almost doesn't exist in rural areas and small towns (Bebtschuk, Smirnova, & Khayretdinov, 2012), where the level of DV is high (Volkova, Lipai, & Wendt, 2015). Needless to say, there is a lack of special education on working with DV in MFT programs at universities with several crisis centers providing workshops and random classes in some universities in major Russian cities. There is a need for developing special curriculum for the MFT programs, where students can learn about the phenomenology of DV and develop appropriate therapeutic skills in working with individuals, couples, and families who have to deal with DV.

DV can include physical, emotional, sexual, economical violent actions, initiated by any of the partners. In this chapter DV will be referred to as *acts of physical violence executed by men toward women*. It is well known that male-to-female violence is one of the most common forms of violence (Montalto, 2016). Some research studies cited in this chapter operate with a term IPV, which will be referred to as violence between people in a close relationship (Timmons, Bryant, Platt, Netko, 2010).

This chapter will present an overview of dominant cultural norms, which endorse DV in modern Russia, addressing social inequalities and providing a rationale for specific treatment for MFT work within DV. Ethical issues in MFT with couples where violence is present will be addressed. Screening, guidelines for conjoint treatment, some therapeutic tools will be provided.

Social Attitudes to Violence in Contemporary Russia

Imagine you are an MFT practitioner in the USA and your client tells you that her husband is planning to kill her. You would probably consult your client, trying to evaluate the risk of the homicide and decide to breach confidentiality, as there would be a risk of death. Then you would probably make a call to police, which would start the investigation. The investigation may end up with a restraining order, so that the perpetrator will be restricted by law in getting close to survivor and her children. However, the situation is drastically different if you work as an MFT practitioner in Russia, which is a country with no DV law. Therefore, if your client tells you that her husband is going to kill her, and hits her every day, and you call the police, "frequently, police will say, we don't' want to deal with this, if he kills her, then we will come" (from a private conversation).

The lack of safety is multiplied by two factors: (a) a limited number of centers, helping victims and survivors of DV; and (b) a low level of education on how to work with victims among the general counseling community. You can hear counselors engaging in the victim blaming, discussing the cycle of violence with both partners, even when one of them is always a perpetrator and another one is constantly a victim. There is a low level of awareness on the matter that a perpetrator may feel empowered and the victim may start feeling guilty for triggering the perpetrator.

The attitudes toward DV are deeply rooted in the minds of Russians and have an impact on the behavior of the perpetrators, victims, and survivors. Stickley, Kislitsyna, Timofeeva, and Vågerö (2008) have researched two aspects of IPV, asking whether violence against women is perceived as a problem and what socio-demographic factors influence this perception. They have also researched if there were specific circumstances which made people justify violence. Researchers provided seven scenarios, in which a husband was beating his wife for a reason. The results have shown that a third of men and over a half of women believed that violence against women is a problem. The most common circumstances to justify violence against women were cases of sexual infidelity. Moreover, both men and women believed that that was a good reason to hit a wife. Therefore, the work of counselors with victims and perpetrators of DV and IPV has to be directed not only at the traumatic consequences of trauma and negotiating the relationship but also at changing attitudes toward violence against women. The work on empowering women and exploring their sense of self-worth is needed.

The idea that "cheating" is more acceptable for men than for women is shown in the Russian folklore, in a proverb, which says, "if they sleep with you, *they abuse us*, but if I sleep with them, *we abuse them*." The meaning of this saying translates as if a husband is having an affair, the whole family benefits from it, but if a wife is having an affair, the whole family suffers and the family boundaries are violated. It is worth noticing that the attitudes, researched by Stickley, Kislitsyna, Timofeeva, and Vågerö (2008) are more prevalent among specific populations; for example, the low level of education makes both male and female being more prone to patriarchal social norms. Additionally, patriarchal social norms are related to the violent behavior (Ozaki & Otis, 2016). Other factors, which exacerbate the relationship and raise the probability of violence in Russia, are economic marginalization and alcohol abuse.

Alcohol Use and Violence in Russia

The level of alcohol consumption in Russia is among the highest in the world, accompanied by tolerance toward drinking, which lessens social control in the society (Pridemore, 2004). However, not all the countries with high alcohol consumption have high rates of violence. Pridemore explains the connection between binge drinking and homicide in Russia, ascribing this relationship to the following factors: (a) preference of strong drinks, such as vodka; (b) less developed bar culture, with drinking happening in private settings (homes and parks); (c) weak formal and social control over binge drinking; (d) a high level of intoxication. Additionally, Cubbins and Vannoy (2005) have shown that frequency of a husband's drinking predicted physical abuse of wives.

According to the meta-analysis performed by Cafferky, Mendez, Anderson and Stith (2016) on 285 studies, substance abuse was significantly related to IPV, with problematic alcohol use measures such as abuse, dependence, drinking problems having stronger correlates than consumption measures such as alcohol use and frequency for the IPV.

The Culture of Oppression and Domestic Violence

Russia has a long history of oppression, which influences the transparency of information concerning DV, as Horne (1999) states, "In the Soviet Union, and now in post-Soviet Russia, there has been a dearth of information, concerning domestic violence, with the majority of crimes unreported to or by the government" (p. 1). Multiple adverse facets of the Russian politics, such as corruption and crime, shaped the culture of violence, making Russia the country with one of the highest homicide rates in the world (Lysova & Shchitov, 2015).

Along with the dearth of information on violence, one would find a paucity of information on oppression in Russian scientific journals; research on deprivation of minorities is banned.

Criteria for oppression in Russia most often include religion, gender identity, sex, nationality and race, age, and ability. DV exists in the culture, where both civilized and uncivilized forms of oppression take place with women being among oppressed individuals, as patriarchal traditions are influential in the modern Russian society. Russian women obtained rights to work without permission of their husbands and to have their own passports in 1917, earlier than women in the USA had these rights (Horne, 1999). However, the tendency to make women equal to men, which emerged after the revolution in 1917, made women obligated to work and to maintain all the housewife responsibilities simultaneously, endorsing double standards for women's role in the society, as depicted by Russian proverb, "I am a horse, and I am a bull, I am a women, I am a man." Putin's presidency is accompanied by a tendency to bring women back at home, give birth and take care of their spouses. The Russian Orthodox Church endorses the restriction for abortions and supports the idea of violence toward children as a disciplinary measure. Additionally, government has cut funding for women's crisis centers (Hardwick, 2014).

Concepts of the Role of Women in Russian Society

The ideal role of a woman for many Russian men would be the one who is compliant and who respects her husband, at the same time being wise to advise her husband – as described by an old Russian saying, "*man is a head, but wife is a neck, head looks where the neck turns.*" One can hear sexist jokes, which lay the foundation for the pyramid of violence: men often say, "Keep silent, woman" and it is considered to be funny. The feminist movement emerges in Russia; however, the majority of Russian women endorse their own oppression by men, and blame feminists for "not being feminine enough and therefore not being real women" (from private conversation).

Meanwhile, sexual equality is seen as central component in prevention of DV as it enables women and men to have equal distribution of power in the relationship. DV is endorsed by male partners claiming to be the head of the household and having the majority of power. Montalto (2016) describes the feminist explanation of DV as embedded into the patriarchal model of society, which makes woman a subordinate, endorsing male domination, therefore the discourse on DV revolves around power, the family structure, with the female role in that structure, aiming at societal change.

DV occurs when one partner feels as having more power than another and wants to reestablish this power again and again. Therefore, in the culture where oppression is supported at the governmental level, it irradiates down to the family unit. The bill, which Amnesty International criticized as an attempt to trivialize domestic violence, was supported by ultra-conservative Russian Parliament female deputies (The law on decriminalization of beating: duma gives green light to beating in families, 2017). These women believe that criminal proceedings must be taken only if there was concussion or broken bones (Russian MPs back bill reducing punishment for domestic violence, 2017).

Thus, Russian women "are caught in a toxic nexus of neoconservative, anti-western, and anti-feminist agendas" (Turbine, 2017). If we add to that the fact that the Russian counseling and psychotherapeutic community is on its way to establishing ethical clinical practice, we will find that the treatment for the victims and survivors of DV may potentially be harmful for the victim as counselors themselves may engage in victim blaming and see partners in conjoint sessions, when intimate terrorism takes place and partners would better be seen individually.

Ethical Considerations

Counseling victims and survivors of domestic violence may be a challenging endeavor for a practitioner in Russia for several reasons: (a) legal – there is no law on domestic violence and no law on counseling and psychotherapy; (b) ethical – counselors tend to engage in victim blaming and try to see the input of a victim in the cycle of violence; many practitioners did not have special courses on ethics in MFT and do not adhere to codes of ethics; (c) educational – one needs to make an effort in finding applicable classes or courses on counseling couples and individuals who have to deal with DV. Currently, Russia has no law which would declare how victims of domestic violence can be protected from the perpetrator. If a counselor evaluates the risk of death for her/his client and reports to police, police may not come and argue, "that it is not in their scope of competence and that partners need to figure everything on their own" (from private conversation).

Client Safety

The absence of the law on the DV and on general counseling practices leads to challenges in protecting a client's safety. Compared to the USA, where the duty to warn and protect is established, Russian counselors decide on their own whether they want to breach the confidentiality to help the victim. The ethical decision making process becomes highly complicated, as after the report would be made to the police, the reaction of the police is unpredictable and can even be aimed at supporting the perpetrator and re-traumatizing the victim.

Family Counselor Education

Many counselors do not obtain proper education on working with victims and survivors of domestic violence and do not usually know how to accurately decide whether the couple should be seen conjointly or separately. The overall stigma towards counseling and psychotherapy stops many couples from seeking counseling, and violent behavior remains under the rug.

The lack of legal regulation and proper education for clinicians is tied to the fact that Russia has no more than 200 crisis centers for more than 130 million people population, unequally distributed across the country. There are regions where women cannot find any help at all. And if you come to Moscow, the capital of Russia, without having special Moscow registration, you will be rejected in getting help at the crisis center in Moscow.

Risks of Re-Traumatization

Victims of DV in Russia are prone to secondary traumatization, which occurs when the victim is followed by skeptical commentaries, accusations of a various kind, pressure to agree to divorce arrangements, which exacerbate the post-separation violence, when partners decide to divorce. Laing (2016) describes the narratives of women who have to deal with the law system when being victims of DV as pressured to keep silence, being controlled and not being able to have the same mother–child relationship they have been having before the divorce (Laing, 2016).

Screening for the Violence in the Family

MFT counselors in Russia need to adhere to screening standards. It is of high importance to screen each couple for the potential presence of domestic violence.

Ghandour, Campbell, and Lloyd (2015) argue that the universal IPV screening is needed for all adolescent girls and women who enter any behavioral care setting, using brief screening tools, which are easy to use and appropriate for diverse populations. Timmons, Bryant, Platt, and Netko (2010) believe that on the intake session an MFT practitioner may have individual time with each partner, so that in case of the intimate terrorism, a victim would be able to share her fears, which may be impossible for a victim if the perpetrator is hearing what she says. Moreover, they provide a list of questions which can be used to screen for the DV in the family. These questions do not need to be asked all at once; a practitioner proceeds with caution and evaluates the risk observing both verbal and nonverbal behavior of partners, checking signs of fear, anxiety, sadness, and grief. Examples of these questions include:

What do arguments between you look like?
When your partner is angry, how does he/she act?
Does your partner get overprotective and jealous?
Have you ever been followed or monitored in any way?
Do you feel that you and your children are in danger?
Is it safe for you to go home?

Timmons, Bryant, Platt, and Netko (2010) recommend starting with open-ended questions and suggest a therapist should weigh the decision to ask questions based on how the client reacts to these questions. These authors also recommend using The Revised Conflict Tactics Scales (CTS2) (Straus, Hamby, Boney-McCoy, & Sugarman, 1996), the Index of Spouse Abuse (ISA) (Hudson & McIntosh, 1981), and the Wife Abuse Inventory (WAI) (Lewis, 1995), which can be problematic for Russian practitioners as these instruments are not translated and validated in Russian. Unfortunately, we could not find any specific instruments to measure spouse abuse. The development of specific instruments screening for DV is needed. These instruments may be used with couples at the intake session to obtain information on the potential markers of violence along with asking screening questions. Once a counselor understands that the DV is taking place in the family, she/he needs to decide whether to continue treatment, and if so, make a decision on the type of treatment.

Choosing the Type of Treatment

Choosing the type of treatment, conjoint or individual therapy would also be a serious question to ask. How can one choose whether to continue seeing partners together or not? And if the couple would be split, does one need to refer both clients to other practitioners? Or refer just one – the perpetrator or the victim? Answers to these questions need to be scrutinized. One of the biggest problems for Russian MFT counselors is seeing the process of solving the DV problems in couples by changing interactions in the relationship. Meanwhile, DV and IPV may be based on control and power, and thus not be reciprocal (Timmons, Bryant, Platt, & Netko, 2010). Johnson's (1995, 2005, 2008) typology of DV includes three types based on control: (a) intimate terrorism or coercive controlling violence, (b) violent resistance, and (c) situational couple violence.

Intimate terrorism or coercive controlling violence is a form of DV in which one partner is systematically being violent toward another partner, using a variety of power and control means, from isolation to harsh corporal violence. Forms of intimate terrorism are depicted in a power and control wheel (Pence & Paymar, 1993). More often this type of DV is used by male against female in the family.

Violent resistance occurs when a victim resists the violence and becomes violent towards a perpetrator. An example would be a Russian woman who had been severely beaten by her husband for years and one day she decides to kill him.

Situational violence is a form of abuse which happens with relatively equal distribution of power and control in a couple. This type of violence is likely to be used by both male and female partners and occurs as a reaction to stressors within a relationship, which partners try to resolve with violence. It is not easy to tell who has more power in the relationship and therefore this is a form of DV which raises a possibility for conjoint treatment.

Therefore, a counselor first assesses the type of the DV, which may be (a) coercive controlling violence, (b) violent resistance, and (c) situational family or couple violence. The following steps would lead to the decision on whether to see the couple conjointly or separately. Armenti and Babcock (2016) discuss the implications of conjoint treatment for IPV, stating that the conjoint treatment approach may only be used with couples with strong evidence of situational violence. That would mean that the violence in the couple won't be motivated with the desire to employ coercive control, there will be a little risk of physical injury, there won't be substance abuse issues involved. Additionally, conjoint treatment should be used when the partners can take responsibility for the violent behavior. However, if the opposite factors are in place, partners should not be seen together.

When a practitioner decides to see the clients separately, he/she must be very careful with preserving the confidentiality of each partner. Although, in MFT practice keeping secrets is not a common practice and some clinicians have the "no secret" policy, in a case of coercive couple violence a practitioner can keep secrets to preserve the confidentiality and safety of the victimized partner.

Substance abuse issues would be another concern for the counselor. Some clinicians tell their clients in cases where DV is involved that they would not continue seeing them if they do not go through the substance abuse evaluation and specific treatment if needed, as abuse decreases impulse control (Stith, McCollum, Rosen, Locke, & Goldberg, 2005) and therapy results may be erased.

In cases of intimate terrorism counselors need to be mindful of helping their clients to develop a safety plan, which victims may use in situations with high risk of lethality. A safety plan may be created in an individual session and describe the individual and social resources, including crisis lines, shelters, close relatives and/or friends a victim may contact in case of emergency. Safety planning may also include advice on preparing the emergency bag, with extra phone, money and documents, baby food, and clothes to escape.

Case Study

Olga, a 24-year-old female and Yuri, a 27-year-old male, made an appointment with Mary, MFT counselor, who was working in private practice in Moscow, Russia. Presented concern was related to the conflicts in the relationship and the desire to enhance sexual life. At the first session, Mary discussed informed consent, explained confidentiality along with the reasons for breaching confidentiality, saying that she would report cases of abuse and violence among family members if those would be of high lethality. At the intake interview Mary noticed that Olga did not talk much and looked shy, with Yuri controlling the conversation and constantly blaming his wife for not satisfying him as a husband. Mary learned that Olga did not work, was financially dependent on her husband, did not have friends as her husband decided that all her friends were unworthy. Yuri also did not like Olga's family and claimed that he "took her out of the dirt" and "made her life Heaven." However, Olga did not look happy as evidenced by her nonverbal behavior.

Mary carefully documented an intake session and decided to consult with the supervisor on how to proceed with the screening of potential DV. Supervisor introduced Mary to the power and control wheel and they figured that Yuri was controlling in most the areas of the wheel. The decision to talk to Olga individually was made. Mary decided to spend individual time with Yuri too, so that in case of him being violent he would not be suspicious and stop Mary from talking to Olga individually.

When Mary asked to have individual time with both partners, Yuri became anxious and said that he did not like the idea as he believed his wife was not smart enough and could confuse the counselor and she liked to make things up. Mary was ethically challenged, as she knew about the ethical principle of honesty and did not want to lie to Yuri; however, she wanted him to let her talk to Olga and she said that she would discuss sexual issues with Olga, which was partially true as she wanted to ask about sexual abuse in the relationship. She did weigh the ethical principles of honesty and do no harm and was sure that her primary goal is to clarify the potential abuse and help the victim.

When Olga and Mary were left in the room together, Olga lifted up her t-shirt and Mary saw a big bruise. Olga put her finger on her lips, showing Mary that she didn't want them to discuss it in the room as she was afraid her husband could hear her. Mary was very challenged. She took a piece of paper and wrote her question on the paper: 1) Does he beat you? Olga wrote yes. The second question Mary wrote was, 2) Does anybody know? Olga wrote, only you. Mary asked a third question: 3) Is there any place you can go? Olga wrote, yes, I can go to my parents. Being concerned with Yuri hearing that there is no conversation in the room, Mary asked Olga some questions about her attitudes towards sexual life in the couple and while she was talking, Mary brought out an outline of a safety plan (Appendix 1) for Olga to review and asked her to fill it in, while she would be talking with her about sexual relationships issues (Appendix 1). Olga took the paper and put it in a secret place. Later next day she called Olga and told her that she was staying with her mother and did contact a crisis center as she was afraid that if she comes back to Olga she could be followed by her husband.

This case scenario shows us a successful work of an MFT counselor, when a victim has enough self-esteem to escape. One of the biggest challenges, however, would be the lack of support from the police and the legal system. As there is no DV law in Russia and the restraining order does not exist, counselors need to discuss all the possible scenarios for a victim if she/he decides to leave the perpetrator. One of the biggest challenges in leaving the abuser is related to the fear that the abuser will follow the victim and will finally kill her. Therefore, in each particular situation, a counselor needs to help the client find as many social support resources as possible. Each Russian counselor needs to have information about crisis centers and shelters which exist in the region where she/he works and where the client lives. Currently, there is only one Internet site which has all existing crisis centers phone numbers which victims may call and get help – http://nasiliu.net/, which is tied to the free mobile phone app https://itunes.apple.com/ru/app/n.n./id1135835949?mt=8 to ask for help. However, the number of crisis centers in the modern Russia is limited and specific programs on developing crisis centers in the country are needed.

Conclusions and Recommendations

This chapter presents a problem of DV in modern Russia, which endorses the culture of oppression at multiple levels, spiraling down to the family unit. Social attitudes toward DV are still close to keeping violence out of mind and out of sight, engaging in victim blaming and supporting the perpetrators, especially male partners, who have the power in the relationship and believe that physical violence may be a way to control the female partner.

Family counselors in Russia do not receive appropriate education in working with victims and survivors of DV and IPV. A low level of ethical awareness among counselors accompanied by the absence of the specific DV law makes working with victims challenging. Practitioners find themselves confused on whether to treat DV couples individually or separately, whether to keep secrets or not, and how to preserve confidentiality. Additionally, many counselors in Russia do not sign informed consent forms and do not explain consent for treatment to their clients, which makes the decisions on breaching the confidentiality even more complex. In terms of legal support, counselors who face the need to report potentially lethal abuse may encounter resistance on behalf of the police, who would decide not to intervene and leave the abuser and the victim to resolve their private matter on their own. This chapter presents most significant ethical concerns in working with DV in MFT along with providing guidelines on how to behave in a situation when a counselor has a suspicion that a DV is taking place. One of the safety tools which counselors in Russia can employ is a safety plan, which helps the victim to become a survivor. Further research is needed to understand the phenomenology of DV in Russia, along with developing strategies to change social attitudes toward DV, empower female population, enhance counselor education, and support the law on DV.

Appendix 1. Safety Plan Template (retrieved from www.thehotline.org/help/path-to-safety/#types)

- Identify your partner's use and level of force so that you can assess the risk of physical danger to you and your children before it occurs.
- Identify safe areas of the house where there are no weapons and there are ways to escape. If arguments occur, try to move to those areas.
- Don't run to where the children are, as your partner may hurt them as well.
- If violence is unavoidable, make yourself a small target. Dive into a corner and curl up into a ball with your face protected and arms around each side of your head, fingers entwined.
- If possible, have a phone accessible at all times and know what numbers to call for help. Know where the nearest public phone is located. Know the phone number to your local shelter. If your life is in danger, call the police.
- Let trusted friends and neighbors know of your situation and develop a plan and visual signal for when you need help.
- Teach your children how to get help. Instruct them not to get involved in the violence between you and your partner. Plan a code word to signal to them that they should get help or leave the house.
- Tell your children that violence is never right, even when someone they love is being violent. Tell them that neither you, nor they, are at fault or are the cause of the violence, and that when anyone is being violent, it is important to stay safe.
- Practice how to get out safely. Practice with your children.
- Plan for what you will do if your children tell your partner of your plan or if your partner otherwise finds out about your plan.
- Keep weapons like guns and knives locked away and as inaccessible as possible.

- Make a habit of backing the car into the driveway and keeping it fueled. Keep the driver's door unlocked and others locked – for a quick escape.
- Try not to wear scarves or long jewelry that could be used to strangle you.
- Create several plausible reasons for leaving the house at different times of the day or night.

References

Armenti, N. A., & Babcock, J. C. (2016). Conjoint treatment for intimate partner violence: A systematic review and implications. *Couple and Family Psychology: Research and Practice, 5*, 109–123. doi:10.1037/cfp0000060.

Bebtschuk, M., Smirnova, D., & Khayretdinov, O. (2012). Family and family therapy in Russia. *International Review of Psychiatry, 24*, 121–127. doi:10.3109/09540261.2012.656305.

Cafferky, B. M., Mendez, M., Anderson, J. R., & Stith, S. M. (2016). Substance use and intimate partner violence: A meta-analytic review. *Psychology of Violence*. doi:10.1037/vio0000074.

Cubbins, L. A., & Vannoy, D. (2005). Socioeconomic resources, gender traditionalism, and wife abuse in urban Russian couples. *Journal of Marriage and Family, 67*, 37–52. doi:10.1111/j.0022-2445.2005.00004.x.

Diakonova-Curtis, D., & Porter, N. (2014). Factors affecting the perceptions of sexual assault of women in Russia. Retrieved from PsycEXTRA Dataset. doi:10.1037/e625292013-001.

Ghandour, R. M., Campbell, J. C., & Lloyd, J. (2015). Screening and counseling for intimate partner violence: A vision for the future. *Journal of Women's Health, 24*, 57–61. doi:10.1089/jwh.2014.4885.

Hardwick, N.-A. (2014). Reviewing the changing situation of women in Russian Society. *E-International Relations Students*. Retrieved from www.e-ir.info/2014/12/20/reviewing-the-changing-situation-of-women-in-russian-society/#_ftnref17.

Hawkins, C. A., & Knox, K. S. (2014). Gender violence and discrimination in Russia: Learning from an American–Russian partnership. *International Social Work, 57*, 511–522. doi:10.1177/0020872814536416.

Horne, S. (1999). Domestic violence in Russia. *American Psychologist, 54*, 55–61. doi:10.1037/0003-066x.54.1.55.

Hudson, W. W., & McIntosh, S. R. (1981). The assessment of spouse abuse: Two quantifiable dimensions. *Journal of Marriage and Family*, 43, 873–888.

Jäppinen, M. (2010). Gender violence and crisis centers for women in Russia. *Social Work and Society International Online Journal*, 8. Retrieved from www.socwork.net/sws/article/view/34/88.

Johnson, M. P. (1995). Patriarchal terrorism and common couple violence: Two forms of violence against women. *Journal of Marriage and the Family, 57*, 283. doi:10.2307/353683.

Johnson, M. P. (2005). The differential effects of intimate terrorism and situational couple violence: Findings from the national violence against women survey. *Journal of Family Issues, 26*, 322–349. doi:10.1177/0192513x04270345.

Johnson, M., P. (2008). *A typology of domestic violence: Intimate terrorism,violent resistance, and situational couple violence*. Boston, MA: Northeastern University Press.

Kitzmann, K. M., Gaylord, N. K., Holt, A. R., & Kenny, E. D. (2003). Child witnesses to domestic violence: A meta-analytic review. *Journal of Consulting and Clinical Psychology, 71*, 339–352. doi:10.1037/0022-006x.71.2.339.

Laing, L. (2016). Secondary victimization: Domestic violence survivors navigating the family law system. *Violence Against Women*. doi:10.1177/1077801216659942.

Lewis, B.Y. (1995). The wife abuse inventory: A screening device for the identification of abused women. *Social Work, 30*(1), 32–35. doi:10.1093/sw/30.1.32.

Lysova, A. V., & Hines, D. A. (2008). Binge drinking and violence against intimate partners in Russia. *Aggressive Behavior, 34*, 416–427. doi:10.1002/ab.20256.

Lysova, A., & Shchitov, N. (2015). What is Russia's real homicide rate? Statistical reconstruction and the "decivilizing process." *Theoretical Criminology, 19*, 257–277. doi:10.1177/1362480614568743.

Montalto, M. (2016). How have academic theories of domestic violence influenced western physical domestic violence treatment programs in recent years? *Journal of Alcoholism & Drug Dependence, 4*. doi:10.4172/2329-6488.1000237.

Ozaki, R., & Otis, M. D. (2016). Gender equality, patriarchal cultural norms, and perpetration of intimate partner violence: Comparison of male university students in Asian and European cultural contexts. *Violence Against Women*. doi:10.1177/1077801216654575.

Pence, E., & Paymar, M. (1993). *Education groups for men who batter: The Duluth model*. New York: Springer.

Prava zenshin – prava cheloveka (2009). Retrieved from: http://nasiliu.net/wp-content/uploads/2016/10/2009_Territoriya-molchaniya.pdf.

Pridemore, W. A. (2004). Weekend effects on binge drinking and homicide: The social connection between alcohol and violence in Russia. *Addiction, 99*, 1034–1041. doi:10.1111/j.1360-0443.2004.00762.x.

Russian MPs back bill reducing punishment for domestic violence. (2017, January 25). *The Guardian*. Retrieved from www.theguardian.com/world/2017/jan/25/russian-mps-bill-reducing-punishment-domestic-violence-rights.

Stickley, A., Kislitsyna, O., Timofeeva, I., & Vågerö, D. (2008). Attitudes toward intimate partner violence against women in Moscow, Russia. *Journal of Family Violence, 23*, 447–456. doi:10.1007/s10896-008-9170-y.

Stith, S.M., McCollum, E. E., Rosen, K. H., Locke, L., & Goldberg, P. (2005). Domestic violence-focused couple treatment. In J. L. Lebow (Ed.), *Handbook of clinical family therapy* (pp. 406–430). New York: John Wiley & Sons.

Straus, M. A., Hamby, S. L., Noney-McCoy, S., & Sugarman, D. B. (1996). The revised conflict tactics scales (CTS2): Development and preliminary psychometric data. *Journal of Family Issues*, 17, 283–316.

Symons, K., Hellemans, S., Van Houtte, M., & Vermeersch, H. (2016). The effect of family violence on sexual victimization among young women. *Journal of Family Violence, 31*, 759–769. doi:10.1007/s10896-016-9803-5.

Taşkale, N., & Soygüt, G. (2016). Risk factors for women's intimate partner violence victimization: An examination from the perspective of the schema therapy model. *Journal of Family Violence, 32*, 3–12. doi:10.1007/s10896-016-9855-6.

The law on decriminalization of beating: duma gives green light to beating in families. (2017, January 19). Amnesty International. Retrieved from https://amnesty.org.ru/ru/2017-01-19-poboi/).

Timmons, S., Bryant, J., Platt, R. A., Netko, D. (2010). Ethical and clinical issues with intimate partner violence. In L. Hecker (Ed.), *Ethics and professional issues in couple and family therapy* (pp. 107–130). Kindle Edition. New York: Routledge.

Turbine, V. (2017). Russia: Decimation of women's human rights in the context of global misogony. *New Eastern Europe*. Retrieved from http://neweasterneurope.eu/articles-and-commentary/2318-russia-decimation-of-women-s-human-rights-in-the-context-of-global-misogyny.

Volkova, O., Lipai, T., & Wendt, S. (2015). Domestic violence in rural arears of Russia and Australia. *International Letters of Social and Humanistic Sciences, 55*, 101–110. doi:10.18052/www.scipress.com/ilshs.55.101.

9

COUNSELING FEMALES IN THE "CAJUN" CULTURE OF SOUTH LOUISIANA

Irene Leblanc

Introduction

The Cajun culture of south Louisiana began with French settlers from western, central France. Under the Treaty of Utrecht, France was forced to cede Acadie to Britain in 1713. These Acadians were then deported to various British colonies along the Atlantic seaboard, including present day Nova Scotia, Canada. These French settlers in Canada were considered a threat by the British amidst the fighting between the British and the French. The Acadians simply wanted neutrality between the British and the French, and did not want to choose sides and fight. This desired, long-lasting neutrality ended in 1754 when the Governor of Canada, Major Charles Lawrence, illegally required those Acadians to sign an oath of absolute loyalty to the King of England, along with renouncing their Catholic religion (LaBorde, n.d.). Those who refused to sign the oath were forced from their families and/or arrested. Entire Acadian colonies were subsequently burned to the ground. This destroyed everything this population of already exiled settlers worked to establish. A mass expulsion then occurred, known as "Le Grande Derangement" or the Great Upheaval. Many families were separated and placed on different ships headed to different states and countries (LaBorde, n.d.).

Arrival in Louisiana

Roughly 4,000 of those exiled Acadians found their way to southern Louisiana, along the fertile land and bayous. The term "Cajun" evolved from the terms Acadie, Acadia, Acadian, and Acadiana. Cajuns arrived in Louisiana as a population, an ethnic group, without a country. Close ties were developed among this group, who only had each other for survival. These Cajuns were content with a simple existence, free to practice their religious beliefs and live their life (Brasseaux, 1992).

"Outsiders" have viewed and still view Cajuns as a singular group of fun, honest, but perhaps ignorant and desperately poor fishermen and trappers (Brasseaux, 1992). This perception may have developed from the non-materialistic nature of the Cajun culture. This culture initially survived by growing and building what the family needed, and then selling what wasn't needed to buy non-essentials. A comfortable lifestyle was all that was desired. An important component of the Cajun culture was and is sharing with others. For example, a garden will most likely produce more than necessary. This surplus is shared with neighbors and anyone who drops in for a visit (Brasseaux, 1992).

This generosity and loyalty extended beyond the family and to the community. This is a protective culture, somewhat enmeshed, and sometimes exclusive. Once you are accepted, the loyalty can extend a lifetime. As readily as one can be accepted, one can also be excommunicated. The general assumption is that people are good and trustworthy, and you will be welcomed – until you prove you are not good and trustworthy. A Cajun person is likely to migrate to the good people, the party, and the festival. These are not difficult to find in south Louisiana.

People generally think of New Orleans when thinking of Louisiana. This includes Mardi Gras, Bourbon Street, and "passing a good time." There is the culture of New Orleans and then there is the culture of Cajun south Louisiana. Both are similar, but drive about one hour southwest of New Orleans, and you will see the difference. The communities become smaller, and the houses (surrounded by sugar cane fields) and yards larger. The party atmosphere is still prevalent; however, the parties are generally in people's homes, rather than a nightclub on Bourbon Street. Any occasion is one to gather people together. The neighbors are invited, as well as any who may just want to "drop in." Along with the best food in the world, it is safe to say there is an impressive amount of alcohol present at gatherings. It is considered rude to not keep a guest's cup and plate full. In this culture, you are showing respect by eating (especially if the host cooked) and perhaps imbibing. Everyone just wants you to join in the fun and the comradery.

In south Louisiana, women generally do the cooking, although a fair number of men participate (and very well). In many homes, you'll find the women in the kitchen, cooking, cleaning, and gossiping, and you'll find the men in the living room watching a LSU or Saints game. It's fair to say that both genders wouldn't likely have it any other way. Most women might say that they do not want the men hanging out in the kitchen – that is their territory.

The term "feminist" is not used very often by Cajun women. It would be unusual to hear a woman over 35 claim to be a feminist. Why is this? Cajun women are generally the head of the household and do not seem to need the title "feminist." No decision is usually made without going through "mama," even though "daddy" may be the breadwinner. You will hear the phrase, "I have to ask mama first" quite often in south Louisiana.

As stated previously, this is a tight-knit, somewhat enmeshed group, sometimes extremely enmeshed group. The interactions and choices are largely interdependent; keeping the community in mind. Cajuns are fiercely loyal to each other, and this is especially true for Cajun women and their friends. This carries over to daughters. It is commonly known that when "boy marries a Cajun girl," they WILL live near her mama. If there is a problem, it is normally discussed with one's mother, sister, and best girlfriends. Outside of this circle, it is no one's business. Even a problem such as problem drinking is expected to remain "in-house." Family can handle the issue with love, tough love, and even gathering others in the circle to help. You are generally taught not to trust professional, outside help. In this culture, for example, if someone passes out drunk in the front yard, you are expected to call that person's family (typically a male member of the family). The police would never be called. This would be disloyal, unless you know the policeman and you know it would be kept under the radar, not an uncommon occurrence.

A Cajun woman who drinks to excess generally suffers the same stigmatization as the rest of North American society. A drunk woman is frowned upon. Reasons for this include the woman being the head-of-household, having children, and "representing" her husband at all times. Women could easily be blamed for the decline of the household, and the break-up of the family if drinking is an issue. Women are primarily responsible for the care of children. Again, this is a responsibility happily accepted, and not easily turned over to outside help. Therefore, a woman who cannot adequately care for her children is viewed in a particularly negative light. The Cajun culture is, in large part, a matriarchal culture. However, a woman is likely also a wife. Her behavior reflects upon, and has the potential to be an embarrassment to, her husband; although he would never say that publicly. A common expectation of this community would be to "get control of your woman." If a woman is drunk, and behaving drunk, her husband, father, and brothers may step in to avoid further embarrassment. This may involve removing your wife, daughter, or sister from a gathering; and quickly. The family will discuss how to proceed, and the problem will be addressed privately. Cajun communities have always been small and "everyone knows everyone." Therefore, a drunk woman at a party will be gossiped about thoroughly. Recovery from this stigmatization is rarely achieved. Once you are labeled an "addict" to any substance, the label sticks. If the family cannot get the situation under control, only then is a professional involved.

There aren't a great number of therapists in small Cajun communities. Everyone would notice your car in the therapist's parking lot! Therefore, to avoid a dual relationship, and town gossip, you may have to drive to a larger city such as Baton Rouge or New Orleans.

A fellow Cajun would understand the gravity of the decision to seek a professional. However, those not from the culture may not know what to expect. There is a lack of research concerning this culture and mental health counseling. The following sections will address Cajun women, problem drinking, and seeking counseling for help with problem drinking.

First, don't be surprised if your client's (identified patient) father, brother, or husband makes the call for an appointment. The client's mother likely directed one of these males to "take care" of the business aspect of scheduling the appointment. This person who makes the initial contact with the mental health professional is likely to be very polite and deferential. Cajuns may find that professional very impressive, but also intimidating. Expect members of the family to respond, "Yes ma'am, and yes sir," even if the therapist is younger.

Therapists are professionals and taught to dress the part. However, it may helpful to take off the jacket, and loosen your tie. Cajuns may walk in and ask if they can relax – perhaps put their feet up. Therapists are taught to meet the client where they are. So, put your feet up as well! You will be appreciated for being yourself. This includes matching the language of the Cajun culture. If your client uses slang, and imperfect English, you may want to rephrase the graduate school, "fancy" words. For example, a word not "innocuous" may garner polite, yet blank stares. Take note of this and use a simpler, yet still explanatory work.

Of course there are highly educated Cajuns, but this population was born of farmers, plantation workers – who learned to provide all for their families. In a manner of minutes, you can find a Cajun who would share heartbreaking stories of a parent, grandparent, or great-grandparent being punished in the schools for speaking Cajun French. Children were hit over the knuckles with a ruler, or made to kneel on dry corn kernels. The abuse became unbearably oppressive, and many parents took their children out of the school system. Many report relatives with a fifth-grade education, or lower. Therefore, even a highly educated Cajun remembers the stories of oppression and discrimination that happened with their loved ones; and wouldn't dare use those "big" words for fear of making anyone feel inferior. A therapist with "airs about them" will not go over as well as a therapist that has a sense of humor and is "down to earth." In the community of addicts, as well as this population, it is appropriate and welcomed to share stories about yourself. This is an effective way to build rapport with those in addiction, as well as the Cajun culture.

Upon arrival at the initial therapy session, you will want to make sure there are enough chairs in your office. You have no idea how many people may decide to attend. You may also want to have a pot of coffee available for the group. This will set a welcoming tone. In most Cajun households, upon arrival, you will be offered fresh coffee. Your client may bring her mama, her sister(s), and her best friend. Of course, this is ideal for a systemic family therapist. For others, this could be an unwelcomed surprise. Many activities from shopping to going to the DMV are done in groups in the Cajun culture. The company is always appreciated. You'll often hear the phrase, "The more the merrier" in south Louisiana.

Building rapport is one the most important components of the therapeutic process. With the Cajun population, it is advisable to build rapport immediately, otherwise you may have a "no-show" for the second session. As mentioned previously, the Cajun circle of trusted family and friends is the most important aspect of life in general. It is not uncommon for women to speak to their female circle of friends and family several times a day. The opinion of this circle is not to be dismissed, but perhaps integrated into the session; without loss of administrative control. For example, the client's mother may seem intrusive with her opinions. The nature of this relationship is to be respected for rapport and progress. If your client's mother is disrespected, the Cajun culture dictates that everyone stand up for and protect the mother; even if she's wrong. This calls on a specific skill set to hear the mother out and compliment her wisdom and devotion. Once the mother feels respected and heard, the therapist could then ask for her help with further ideas. When rapport is established, as with the previous example, the therapist will be supported and the mother will likely insist everyone support and listen to the therapist's suggestions. At this point, don't be surprised if a gift is brought or homemade food. These are signs of love and acceptance in the Cajun culture. If the food is homemade, it is advisable to have some while the session is occurring. In terms of rapport building, and being accepted, there is no more powerful response to a Cajun client than to enjoy their food.

At some point, the therapist may utilize couple's therapy, as a concomitant to "family therapy." The enmeshed, closed system of the Cajun culture should still be considered. The loyalty runs deep and this isn't always healthy loyalty. The husband may want to learn new, and healthier ways, but the wife's family will likely have a strong influence.

The therapist may benefit from asking the couple, "Who is triangulated into the problems currently experienced?" This provides information regarding outside influences on the marriage. For example, the wife may state that discussing personal issues with mother, or others, is quite a normal occurrence. Drinking with family and friends may be a part of the relationship for the client. Females identify alcohol as the primary substance abused across all cultures in the United States (SAMHSA, 2011). You may have a husband state that his wife or partner spends too much time at her mother's house. His mother-in-law may spend a great deal of time in his home, uninvited. This mom likely has her own key, and doesn't bother knocking on the door. Those outside of the culture may find this rude and intrusive. In south Louisiana, this is an everyday occurrence.

Case Example

Consider the case study of Christine, a somewhat extreme example of dating/ marrying a Cajun woman:

> Christine is the middle child of five. She is extremely loyal to both parents. Christine has had no friends throughout her life. The few times she attempted to socialize, the friends were eventually pushed away. Christine always seemed to find a reason not to like them. The other four siblings have some semblance of a social life, and all married. Christine had one short-lived marriage, that was contentious and not loving. She has a long history of jealousy toward her siblings, in particular her younger sister (the star of the family).
>
> All romantic relationships end dramatically with the boyfriend being the one to call off the relationship. Her boyfriends often report her fear of abandonment, and overly dramatic nature to be the reason for the break-up. Christine often exaggerates to bolster her own sense of importance, or just to watch the drama unfurl. This day-to-day drama is relayed to daily visits to home, primarily to have long conversations with her mother that are solely negative in nature, with no positive solution discussed. Both mother and daughter seem to provide a purpose for each other, with Christine being willing to take on the role of "scapegoat" and sacrifice her life to bolster and maintain the relationship with her mother. The mother, as with most Cajun families, is the most powerful family member. Christine is considered the "best" child, due to her sacrificing what most would consider healthy behaviors; a relationship, hobbies, and friendships. In this family, being "healthy" is not necessarily encouraged. It threatens the carefully constructed closed system. No one is allowed in and no one is allowed out. This is a covert directive that no one would likely acknowledge as true. After all, it's good to go to college and have healthy outside relationships. However, to do so means threatening the homeostasis of the family, with ensuing efforts to covertly or overtly avert this behavior. In this particular family, two of the five children were "disloyal," meaning they accepted outside relationships and beliefs; and were willing to set appropriate boundaries. Although happier in general, there was a high price to pay for this "disloyalty." Emotional cut-offs are common when homeostasis is threatened. The two siblings that chose "happiness" are the only two siblings out of the five that speak to each other regularly.

An intervention with Christine, the subject of the case study, is twofold. First, what is that Christine wants to accomplish in therapy, given her cultural boundaries, and history? Second, is Christine willing to have others involved in treatment? Given her self-reported history of exaggeration and propensity for drama, other family members could provide more accurate information. Upon signing a consent for release of information, the therapist is able to speak to Christine's four siblings. Christine does not consent to her mother being involved, as the mother is bedridden due to a recent cancer diagnosis. Christine reports she wants to improve her familial relationships with her siblings and wants a long-lasting romantic relationship.

Three of the four siblings were contacted and reported largely the same story. All report a long history of extreme drama that includes threats of suicide attempts, cutting, fabricated illness (MS), and even a false report of being raped. The report includes Christine doing "anything to garner attention and to wreak havoc." One of the siblings, Marie, reported that their parents believe Christine and feel sorry for her. Marie stated that Christine will not want this dynamic changed by her parents knowing the truth about her "extreme lies." Of the three siblings, Marie reports being the only one that has been willing to break the rules of the family and mostly go her own way. Marie is the most resistant to "falling for Christine's narcissistic charm again."

All three siblings report a relationship with Christine that ranges from limited contact to no contact. None of the siblings are willing to participate in treatment, as they expressed the likelihood that Christine is also using the therapy process as a further excuse for her behaviors and to gain more attention. Three of siblings (excluding Marie) stated they are willing to accept continued phone calls from the therapist.

A specific intervention for Christine would be to make the covert overt, and to address the issues introduced by the siblings. In addition to conjoint family therapy, group therapy for Christine may be useful, in that others in a group therapy setting could point out specific behaviors in "real time" and address these behaviors on the spot. The therapist could assign "accountability" as well for the client, and have her begin (slowly) being honest about issues, and attempt to make amends. Follow-up sessions may include the siblings to discuss any progress and remaining issues. These interventions should be framed with the mother of the family in mind – perhaps as a means of making the mother happier in seeing her children function better as a family. Remember, the mother is the glue in the Cajun family.

Boundaries in the Cajun culture are somewhat blurred; some may state there are no defined boundaries. As stated previously, when boy marries Cajun girl, he may have to defer to his mother-in-law. Mothers are very powerful in the Cajun culture. This lends itself to a cross-cultural relationship – with a need for increased knowledge and education. The opportunity to compromise presents itself, along with setting boundaries.

The Cajun community as a closed, and at times "enmeshed" culture in terms of social support traces its origins to the "Le Grande Derangement" of the Cajuns, when members of the Cajun community relied exclusively upon each other for support.

Female social relationships in general are seen as paramount to well-being and general happiness (Canfield, 2018). This is especially true in the Cajun culture. When addressing addiction, decreased positive social support is a problem in active addiction, (Tyler, 2008; Buchanan & Latkin, 2008). Social support is important to both males and females; however, females tend to rely on these connections to a greater degree (Sutherland, 2009) and are much more likely to reach out for help than males (Koos et al., 2014). In a close-knit society, as the Cajun culture, this may involve several visits or phone calls a day to family and friends. These relationships are viewed as important to general coping and wellness. Building these social networks is important to treatment outcomes and contributes to long-term sobriety (Knight, Wallace, Joe, & Logan, 2001). Females who improve social support, while avoiding negative social interactions, demonstrate improved treatment outcomes (Ellis, Bernichon, Yu, Roberts, & Herrell, 2004). Further, positive social support provides momentum for improved wellness (West, Hosie, & Zarski, 1987). The therapist must then navigate possible negative relationships within the Cajun family. This can be challenging. Perhaps the client engages in drinking with family or friends that contribute to the problem drinking. Settings boundaries in this area would require a delicate balance of not offending family or friends. You may be presenting ideas never before attempted.

Systemic family therapy skills can be utilized in many ways to introduce boundaries and avoidance of triggering situations. The one-down method espoused by family therapist John Weakland may be useful. Bringing in family and friends to "help" would be a respectful, engaging method. Setting boundaries could be presented as an issue the client is having, and needs help. If the therapist has established rapport, family and friends will likely show enthusiasm in helping their loved one. After all, the client's family and friends know the client better than anyone. This respect of their knowledge, as with most, would set the stage for introducing new boundaries. For example, if drinking is a problem while visiting, family member could offer alternatives. Perhaps home visits, especially when new to recovery, could be limited to morning coffee. These important connections can remain, just in an adjusted context.

While maintaining these connections, positive connections can also be developed outside of the immediate circle of family and friends. This can be accomplished with various Alcoholics Anonymous meetings, church groups, etc. Family and friends can be encouraged to attend these activities, to avoid fear of the client being disloyal to the relationship "system." Remember, the Cajun culture can be enmeshed and closed off to outsiders, so the "primary" relationships must be respected.

The distrust of outsiders exists to this day, based on the historic, systematic stigmatization of Cajuns. Cajuns have been treated and are still sometimes treated as backward, uneducated, and simple people. Many Cajuns recall their parents and grandparents comfortably speaking Cajun French, but fumbling with speaking or reading English. This often leads to feeling the stigmatization of being from a "lower" culture.

In the Cajun culture, as with general society, females experience more stigmatization than males (White & Kilbourne, 2006). This often leads to females not seeking treatment for problem drinking, due to feeling less worthy of treatment and care from others (Carrière, 2008; Back et al., 2006)). In the United States, females experience harsher social attitudes, and are stigmatized and vilified for their addiction more than males (Brady & Randall, 1999). This is no different in the Cajun culture. Females may even take more precautions to be secretive when in active addiction, given the close nature of the Cajun culture. Everyone in community will likely know if there is a struggle with problem drinking.

Patriarchal societies often approve of males drinking, but women are only expected to drink in moderation (Dragišić, 2016). Although the Cajun culture can be matriarchal in nature, there remains an expectation to uphold family values and represent your husband in a respectable fashion. As referenced earlier, females traditionally care for and maintain the family; therefore, female drinking is considered a more serious problem that can cause family decline (Williams & Sternthal, 2010).

Of course, many Cajun females work outside the home. Normally, the responsibilities in the home with husband and children remain. It is not unusual for many of these women to work a full day outside the home, to return home and cook dinner and tend to children (usually by choice). Having children is generally a double-edged sword to an addict. Children can motivate one to hide addiction at a more expert level, and also provide motivation for treatment and recovery (Darke et al., 2007). Once treatment is initiated, females are more likely to sustain abstinence than men, which indicates receptiveness to effective treatment (Darke et al., 2007).

Effective treatment is culturally sensitive, as well as sensitive to the person's system of relationships. Professional women in this culture likely have an additional burden to keep problem drinking under control. The secretive nature of this addiction would seem to take its toll over time, given the added professional duties. This means holding it together while at work and home. In time, this stress accumulates, possibly leading to increased consumption of alcohol, with ensuing consequences. Oksanen (2013) reports that "addiction has more severe consequences to the professional career of women" (p. 136). There will likely be less understanding for women. These differences are consistently more harmful for females than for males (Oksanen, 2013; Sallmann, 2010). Females could benefit from these differences being addressed in treatment. Treatment that addresses female-specific issues is hypothesized to positively correlate with treatment retention and treatment outcomes (Koos et al., 2014). Positive social support is positively correlated to health and well-being in all cultures (Cohen, 2004). Improved overall wellness leads to decreased alcohol abuse and relapse (The National Institute on Drug Abuse [NIDA], 2016).

Researchers identify females as more vulnerable to family dysfunction, depression, and feelings of shame and guilt over their addiction (Finkelstein, 1996). Relapse rates among substance abusers, male or female, is estimated to be between 40% and 60% (NIDA, 2014). An exact percentage is unknown, particularly given the secretive nature of substance abuse. There is an increased exposure to unfavorable social factors with female substance abusers (Chatham, Hiller, Rowan-Szal, Joe, & Simpson, 1999; Chiang et al., 2007). Tracy et al. (2012) determined in their study that many substance abusing females had low incomes, lived in poor neighborhoods, and experienced numerous factors that could complicate access to treatment and supportive services. During a follow-up interview, Tracy et al. (2012) also observed a decrease in social quality of life, which may "indicate a vulnerable time point for women in treatment during which they may have extricated themselves from some substance-involved social relationships but not replaced them with more appropriate social outlets; social support or network interventions might be timely and relevant at this point in time as well" (p. 247).

In the United States, there are many factors researched and reported specifically for females. Some of these factors include; (1) overall, females typically have less education and employment options/skills (Chen et al., 1998), (2) studies have demonstrated that early drug and alcohol use among females is associated with lower levels of educational attainment (Dryden, 2012), and (3) early alcohol use and alcohol dependence possibly impede later educational attainment (Grant et al., 2012). Additional reasons for this impediment include cognitive and motivational effects which begin with early alcohol use/dependence, and this can limit academic and employment success (Grant et al., 2012). In most cultures, education is encouraged and highly valued. However, you may find the opposite in the Cajun culture. Many young people follow in their parents' footsteps by working in oil-related or farming jobs (for example). This is hard work that pays well, but doesn't always require higher education. A perception can be that with higher education, you are being disloyal to the system (Cajun culture), and may leave the system. The Cajun culture is often a closed system, with a lack of new ideas or people allowed. Of course, there are exceptions, but this is a common occurrence in this culture. An addiction to alcohol can serve to keep one embedded in the current situation, healthy or not. Therefore, in a culture that is traditionally closed and enmeshed, the motivation to break trends might be undesired and discouraged by others.

Females, in the United States, report a higher dysfunctional family of origin (Chen et al., 1998). Moreover, females from an addictive family of origin have a high likelihood that they may grow up suffering with lifelong psychological and emotional problems (Tracy et al., 2012). The National Institute on Alcohol Abuse and Alcoholism (2002) published a study (Grant et al., 2012) which indicated that roughly 25% of children in the United States will grow up in an addictive home. Other researchers have also concluded that this 1 in 4 ratio is an appropriate estimate (Tracy et al., 2012). The close Cajun culture would dictate that these problems remain "in-house" as long as possible. If the dysfunction is not controlled, the entire community will likely become aware of the issues.

In a study conducted by Ponder and Slate (2010), graduate students (N = 129) in counseling and psychology programs were studied to determine the extent to which addiction was present in their family of origin. The females in this study reported a higher percentage of family-of-origin alcoholism and drug addiction (Ponder & Slate, 2010). The percentage of females in the Cajun culture is unknown. However, given the "festival" culture of south Louisiana, the number could be at or above the national average. This indicates, potentially, a long history of family dysfunction as well as addictive behaviors which garner stigmatization.

Stigmatization is a mutually consensual relationship between the individual and society. Each society has its own cultural norms for what constitutes social support, as well as stigmatization. Social norms in south Louisiana dictate loyalty to the family, and friends that are like family. Decisions are made with loved ones in mind, sometimes with the self as a secondary consideration.

Stigmatization is a reality in the Cajun culture, as well as society in general. Females are mothers, with no more important task than caring for the family. Any compromises in this endeavor will result in that person being "marked." Unfortunately, no matter how "good" the person is, there will be a mark of stigmatization for the negative behavior. One of the most disturbing things that can happen to a woman is the loss of custody of her children. To choose a drug over one's children is the considered by some to be the gravest of sins, and the stigma is long-lasting, if not forever. In small south Louisiana towns, this stigma can persist for generations.

Stigmatization is important to consider because it affects social support. When stigmatization factors in, perceived or otherwise, social support and overall wellness decreases. In a recent study by the author (Canfield, 2018), 232 females, in the general US population, with a substance use disorder completed three surveys addressing wellness, social support, and stigmatization. These surveys were the Perceived Wellness Survey (PWS) (Adams, Bezner, & Garner, & Woodruff, 1998), the Multidimensional Scale of Perceived Social Support (MSPSS) (Zimet, Dahlem, Zimet, & Farley, 1988), and the Perceived Stigmatization of Addiction Scale (PSAS) (Luoma et al., 2010). Participants filled out these three surveys, as well as a demographic form. The purpose of this study was to determine the role of social support as a mediator between stigmatization and wellness. More specifically, the hypothesis was that with increased social support, there is decreased stigmatization and increased wellness. Conversely, with decreased social support, there is increased stigmatization and decreased wellness. The results from this study were significant. Social support was determined to completely mediate the relationship between stigmatization and wellness. Final analyses determined that with positive social support, perceived stigmatization is decreased, and there is an increase in overall wellness. Further, stigmatization is correlated with wellness. These results support the information provided in this chapter. Social support is important in addiction, but it must be positive social support. This would mean, for Cajun females specifically, to set boundaries with current sources of social support, and to possibly eliminate sources of negative social support. Negative social support would be defined as those who do not support boundaries needed for sobriety and wellness. This may sound harsh, but for addicts, it becomes an issue of survival.

Implications and Recommendations

The implications are significant for the Cajun culture, and females in particular. Females place a high value on personal relationships, more so than males. The Cajun culture is known for being close, and sometimes enmeshed. Females normally stay close to home, even when married. Friends and family are normally contacted several times a day; sometimes just to discuss mundane details of life. Without a positive support system, females suffer increased depression, anxiety, and decreased overall wellness. Problem drinking is sometimes a method of self-medicating. It can be done anytime, with complete privacy. The combination of poor coping skills, lack of positive social connections, and perceived stigmatization, is a dangerous combination. It is particularly dangerous in a small social community where acceptance is not automatic, and everyone knows everyone. Those who grow up Cajun consider themselves to be pretty lucky. The friendliest people live there, once you get to know them. There is always a party or gathering somewhere, and everyone wants to feed you the best food in the world. However, this isn't the case for 100% of the Cajun population. Addiction is a problem of isolation, secrecy, and loneliness. These problems tend to exacerbate as the addiction worsens. This results in a particular problem in this culture. Seeing a therapist is a huge step, and a risky one. Reputations are risked, as well as being emotionally cut-off from the family and/or friends. For therapists, education for your clients is important in the following ways; (1) to understand the progressive nature of addiction, (2) to understand that it is much more difficult to address addiction and sobriety on your own, and (3) to understand (possibly) new concepts such as boundary setting and reframing of addiction. Boundary setting may prove to be especially difficult in the Cajun culture. If not handled delicately, it could be viewed as disrespectful. One method is to invite the "powerful" people in the system to participate in therapy and "help" the therapist. It would be a much longer process without this help. Further, using this method, you are helping your client achieve their goals, without having to fight the system. A Cajun female would not likely be receptive to challenging the system.

Conclusions and Recommendations

This is a loving and loyal group of people. Have them join you in this process. Most importantly, remember that this is a culture that, despite efforts over the last 250 years to destroy the culture, has survived as a very distinct group. The Cajun traditions have survived, and do not seem likely to change. You are more likely to change the course of a Cajun family's dysfunction by joining this family, rather than going against its flow. Remember to take off your shoes, loosen your tie, and enjoy whatever food is brought to the party (or therapy session).

References

Adams, T. B., Bezner, J., Garner, L., & Woodruff, S. (1998). Construct validation of the Perceived Wellness Survey. *American Journal of Health Studies*, 14(4), 212.

Back, S. E., Brady, K. T., Sonne, S. C., & Verduin, M. L. (2006). Symptom improvement in co-occurring PTSD and alcohol dependence. *The Journal of Nervous and Mental Disease*, 194(9), 690–696.

Bateson, G., Jackson, D. D., Haley, J., & Weakland J. (1956). Toward a theory of schizophrenia. *Behavioral Science*, 1(4), 251–264.

Brady, K. T., & Randall, C. L. (1999). Gender differences in substance use disorders. *Addictive Disorders*, 22, 241–252.

Brasseaux, C. A. (1992). *Acadian to Cajun: Transformation of a People, 1803–1877*. Jackson: University Press of Mississippi.

Buchanan, A. S., & Latkin, C. A. (2008). Drug use in the social networks of heroin and cocaine users before and after drug cessation. *Drug and Alcohol Dependence*, 96(3), 2008, 286–289.

Canfield, I. (2018). The impact of social support, stigmatization upon the wellness of females diagnosed with a substance use disorder. (Unpublished doctoral dissertation). Department of Counselor Education, College of Education, Florida Atlantic University, Boca Raton, Florida.

Carrière, G. L. (2008). Linking women to health and wellness: Street outreach takes a population health approach. *International Journal of Drug Policy,* 19(3), 205–210. doi:10.1016/j.drugpo.2008.03.006.

Chatham, L. R., Hiller, M. L., Rowan-Szal, G. A., Joe, G. W., & Simpson, D. D. (1999). Gender differences at admission and follow-up in a sample of methadone maintenance clients. *Substance Use and Misuse*, 34(8), 1137–1165.

Chen, C. K., Shu, L. W., Liang, P. L., Hung, T. M., & Lin, S. K. (1998). Drug use patterns and gender differences among heroin addicts hospitalized for detoxification. *Changgeng Yi Xue Za Zhi,* 21(2), 172–178.

Chiang, S., Chan, H., Chang, Y., Sun, H., Chen, W. J., & Chen, C. (2007). Psychiatric comorbidity and gender difference among treatment-seeking heroin abusers in Taiwan. *Psychiatry and Clinical Neurosciences,* 61(1), 105–111. doi:10.1111/j.1440 1819.2007.01618.x.

Cohen, S. (2004). Social relationships and health. *American Psychologist,* 59(8), 676–684. doi:10.1037/0003-066X.doi:59.8.676.

Darke, S., Ross, J., Mills, K. L., Williamson, A., Havard, A., & Teesson, M. (2007). Patterns of sustained heroin abstinence amongst long-term, dependent heroin users: 36

months findings from the Australian Treatment Outcome Study (ATOS). *Addictive Behaviors,* 32(9), 1897–1906. doi:10.1016/j.addbeh.2007.01.014.
Dragišić, S. (2016). Alcohol use: social aspect, gender differences and stigmatization. *Alcoholism & Psychiatry Research*, 52(1), 51–64.
Dryden, J. (2012). Early substance use linked to lower educational achievement. Retrieved from http://source.wustl.edu/2012/05/early-substance-use-linkined-to-lower0educational-achievement.
Ellis, B., Bernichon, T., Yu, P., Roberts, T., & Herrell, J. M. (2004). Effect of social support on substance abuse relapse in a residential treatment setting for women. *Evaluation and Program Planning,* 27 (2), 213–221. doi:10.1016/j.evalprogplan.2004.01.011.
Finkelstein, N. (1996). Using the relational model as a context for treating pregnant and parenting chemically dependent women. *Journal of Chemical Dependency Treatment*, 6(5), 23–44.
Grant, J. D., Scherrer, J. F., Lynskey, M. T., Agrawal, A., Duncan, A. E., Haber, J. R., Heath, A. C., & Bucholz, K. K. (2012). Associations of alcohol, nicotine, cannabis, and drug use / dependence with educational attainment: Evidence from Cotwin – control analysis. *Alcoholism: Clinical and Experimental Research,* 36(8), 1412–1420. doi:10.1111/j.1538–0277.2012.01752.x.
Knight, D. K., Wallace, G. L., Joe, G. W., & Logan, S. M. (2001). Change in psychosocial functioning and social relations among women in residential substance abuse treatment. *Journal of Substance Abuse*, 13(4), 533–547.
Koos, E., Brand, M., Rojas, J., & Li, J. (2014). Sex-specific substance abuse treatment for female healthcare professionals: Implications. *Southern Medical Journal,* 107(1), 28–33. doi:10.1097/SMJ.doi:0000000000000049.
LaBorde, J. (n.d.). A short history of the Acadians and Cajuns. Retrieved from www.medschool.lsuhsc.edu/genetics_center/louisiana/article_cajunhistory.htm.
Luoma, J. B., O'Hair, A. K., Kohlenberg, B. S., Hayes, S. C., & Fletcher, L. (2010). The development and psychometric properties of a new measure of perceived stigma toward substance users. *Substance Use & Misuse,* 45(1–2), 47–57. doi:10.3109/10826080902864712.
National Institute on Drug Abuse (NIDA). (2014). Women who receive gender-specific substance abuse treatment have a greater chance of employment. Retrieved from www.drugabuse.gov/news-events/news-releases/2014/12/women-who-receive-gender-specific-substance-abuse-treatment-have-greater-chance-emp.
Oksanen, A. (2013). Female rock stars and addiction in autobiographies. *Nordic Studies in Alcohol and Drugs,* 30(1–2), 123–140. doi:10.2478/nsad-2013-0009.
Ponder, F. T., & Slate, J. R. (2010). Family of origin addiction patterns amongst counseling and psychology students. Forum on Public Policy. Published by the Forum on Public Policy. Retrieved from https://files.eric.ed.gov/fulltext/EJ903827.pdf.
Sallmann, J. (2010). Going hand-in-hand: Connections between women's prostitution and substance use. *Journal of Social Work Practice in the Addictions,* 10(2), 115–138. doi:10.1080/15332561003730155.
Substance Abuse and Mental Health Services Administration (SAMHSA). (2011). Center for Behavioral Health Statistics and Quality. Individuals admitted to substance abuse treatment have less education than the general U.S. population. Retrieved from www.samhsa.gov.
Sutherland, R. (2009, May). Basic science. *Breast Cancer Online*, 1–2. doi:10.1017/S1470903109990253.

Tracy, E. M., Laudet, A., Min, M., Kim, H., Brown, S., Jun, M., & Singer, L. (2012). Prospective patterns and correlates of quality of life among women in substance abuse treatment. *Drug and Alcohol Dependence,* 124(3), 242–249. doi:10.1016/j.drugalcdep.2012.01.010.

Tyler, K. A. (2008). Social network characteristics and risky sexual and drug related behaviors among homeless young adults. *Social Science Research,* 37(2), 673–685. doi:10.1016/j.ssresearch.2007.09.004.

West, J. D., Hosie, T. W., & Zarski, J. J. (1987). Family dynamics and substance abuse: A preliminary study. *Journal of Counseling and Development*, 65, 487–490. doi:10.1002/j.1556-6676.1987.tb00762.x.

White, W., & Kilbourne, J. (2006). American women and addiction: A cultural double bind. *Counselor, (7)*3, 46–51.

Williams, D. R., & Sternthal, M. (2010). Understanding racial-ethnic disparities in health: Sociological contributions. *Journal of Health and Social Behavior,* 51(1) (Suppl), S15–S27. doi:10.1177/0022146510383838.

Zimet, G. D., Dahlem, N. W., Zimet, S. G., & Farley, G. K. (1988). The multidimensional scale of perceived social support. *Journal of Personality*, 52(1), 30–41.

10

MATE SELECTION COUNSELING FOR CHINESE WOMEN

Ruoxi Chen, Stephen E. May, Jarodd W. Hundley, and Jason P. Austin

Introduction

Mate selection is frequently studied by social psychologists, but rarely by family counselors. Yet the values and expectations of young adults in choosing a spouse may affect their future relationship in myriad ways. Insights into how young adults develop and adjust their mate selection criteria and how different cultural contexts shape this process may guide family therapists and relationship educators in helping individuals navigate this important and often confusing process, and may also inform the therapist in planning therapy to address present relationship issues. This chapter examines key cultural scripts particularly relevant to Chinese women's mate selection process, and demonstrates how therapists may use selected therapy techniques when working with Chinese women struggling with this process.

The Cultural Context for Chinese Women's Mate Selection

The process of finding a mate and the development of relationships in China have evolved greatly over the last century. Chinese young adults have traditionally been expected to marry young and produce offspring soon after marriage. Most Chinese women are married by the ages of 35 to 39 and fewer than 5% of men remain single (Ji & Yeung, 2014). In traditional Chinese marriages, parents would arrange the marriage in advance for the mutual benefit of the families, and neither men nor women were free to choose their partner (Jung, 1999). The primary function of marriage for Chinese individuals was to continue the family line, retain a connection with the family's ancestors, and care for the elders of the family. Whereas the mate selection process for individuals in the Western cultures focuses more on love and connectedness, the mate selection process in China has centered more on conforming to society and has placed great importance on traditional family values (e.g., Dion & Dion, 1993; Hu, Sze, Chen, & Fang, 2015; Toro-Morn & Sprecher, 2003; Zhang & Kline, 2009). Nonetheless, as a result of recent social, economic, and political development, a significant shift has occurred in Chinese marriages and family values. Noticeable changes include the increased importance of love to relationships, greater independence and increased power for women, and higher divorce rates (Hu et al., 2015).

Currently, Chinese individuals' mate selection process is also significantly affected by the country's imbalanced sex ratio, which will exert a greater effect on this process in the near future. China's one-child policy, which was introduced in 1979 and discontinued recently, had resulted in a disproportionately high number of male children compared to females, as female fetuses were more likely to be aborted for the chance to conceive a male child. The consequences of the dramatic imbalance of men and women in China and the insufficient number of marriage-age single Chinese women has increased the probability of women marrying before the age of 25 (Trent & South, 2011).

Despite the imbalanced sex ratio at birth and the resulting lack of marriage-age single Chinese women in the mate selection market, Chinese women still face unique challenges in mate selection. Consider the popular term "leftover women," which refers to unmarried Chinese women in their late 20s to 30s who are often college educated and stigmatized as picky and selfish (To, 2013). Ji (2015) explored how these "leftover women" negotiated the often conflicting goals of finding a mate and having a career, and found parental pressure, the gender double standard of aging, forced socioeconomic hypergamy, and tensions arising from gender ideology as recurring themes of these women's experiences. Another phenomenological study similarly found that core meanings of being a single Chinese woman over the age of 30 included awareness of the advantages (e.g., freedom, autonomy, and independence) and disadvantages (e.g., loneliness and pressure to marry) of being single, ambiguous feelings toward marriage, and adjustments to being single (e.g., learning to face inquiries about marital status skillfully, acclimatizing to being alone) (Wang & Abbott, 2013).

Furthermore, women's marriage market shrinks much more rapidly than men's due to age, because unmarried older men are more likely to marry younger women than they are women in their own age cohort (England & McClintock, 2009). Additionally, post high school education seems to affect Chinese men and women's mate selection differently, prompting men to marry earlier while delaying Chinese women's mate selection process (Jones & Gubhaju, 2009; Tian, 2013). The combination of Chinese women's enhanced economic independence and mate selection criteria and the cultural prescriptions of women marrying up and men marrying down further complicates both genders' mate selection success (Chen, 2016).

Given the cultural scripts noted above, many Chinese women – especially those who are educated, in their late 20s or older, and less willing to compromise on their mate selection criteria – may experience the mate selection process as extremely challenging. Furthermore, their mate selection struggles may have significant ramifications for their relationships with their family of origin, career development, self-perceptions, and future marital relationship.

Culturally Sensitive Approaches for Counseling Chinese Women on Mate Selection Issues

Chinese clients tend to prefer a therapist who assumes the role of expert or teacher, and expect the therapist to actively intervene in therapy (Epstein et al., 2012). At the same time, younger Chinese adults who are more influenced by Western cultures might be further receptive to a more collaborative therapeutic approach (Chen, 2012; Toro-Morn & Sprecher, 2003). Taking into consideration the aforementioned cultural scripts, the following concepts and techniques may be well suited for helping Chinese women navigate the mate selection process, which can be stressful and demoralizing.

Promoting Differentiation

Of particular relevance to Chinese women's mate selection experience is the concept of differentiation, which refers to individuals' ability to separate their thoughts from emotions and to separate their own thoughts and feelings from those of others (Kerr & Bowen, 1988). A well-differentiated person is likely to be more flexible and less reactive. Conversely, a low level of differentiation may prompt anxiety, marital dissatisfaction, and emotional reactivity (Miller, Anderson, & Keals, 2004). Chinese individuals' mate selection pressures stem heavily from parental influences, helping them differentiate from their family of origin might be particularly beneficial.

To promote clients' differentiation, therapists might use genograms to help identify dysfunctional intergenerational patterns in clients' family and to enhance their awareness of such patterns and their potential impact on the clients' relationships (Kerr & Bowen, 1988). For instance, if a woman marries someone whose perceived value is lower than hers, she may experience self-doubt and negative social consequences for opposing the hypergamy norm (e.g., her parents may express disappointment in her or her peers may make snide remarks about her choices). Therapists can use genograms to introduce further insights into clients' mate selection process and discuss with clients; for instance, mate selection traits particularly valued in their family of origin and how such family legacies may have shaped their own approach to mate selection (McGoldrick, Gerson, & Shellenberger, 1999).

The therapist may also encourage clients to utilize "I" statements to take more ownership of their mate selection process. For instance, many Chinese young adults may state their mate selection goal and criteria as: "My parents/family would like me to marry someone who is …" Therapists might help these clients distinguish external mate selection criteria from their own desires, and enhance their ability to tolerate anxiety transferred from their family of origin without overreacting.

Drawing Boundaries

With a higher level of differentiation, clients might also be able draw clearer and more functional boundaries in relation to their extended family to help them assert their autonomy in mate selection. External influences from the media, parents, and peers are significant sources of Chinese young adults' mate selection perceptions and criteria (Chen & Austin, 2017). Many cultural scripts, such as filial piety, can make Chinese individuals feel that they must accept their parents' influence on their mate selection choices. Moreover, Chinese parents' intimate involvement in their adult children's mate selection is commonly practiced and normalized, with many parents going to such lengths as frequenting parks with photographs of their daughters in hopes of finding them a suitable mate (Ji, 2015). As such, Chinese individuals may also benefit from assistance with establishing clearer boundaries between themselves and their family of origin to make more independent mate selection decisions.

Because parental involvement and interferences tend to be normalized in the Chinese cultural context and their negative impact on Chinese individuals' mate selection process tends to be unacknowledged, therapists can help clients identify diffuse boundaries with parents and extended family members (Minuchin & Fishman, 1981). The therapist should clarify that they are not advising clients to blanketly reject parents' influences or to sever ties with their family of origin. Such actions may in fact create a dysfunctional boundary. Instead, the therapist should help these clients develop healthier boundaries that honor parents' well-intentioned and culturally accepted expression of concern for their adult children's well-being, but that nonetheless enables the clients to assert their autonomy. Because it is unlikely that these Chinese women will enroll in therapy with their parents to process their mate selection struggles, the therapist might consider incorporating techniques such as the "empty chair technique" (Greenberg, Rice, & Elliott, 1993) to help clients practice asserting their mate selection choices without becoming overly reactive.

Developing an Alternative Narrative

The use of narrative therapy has benefits with clients of different cultures and ethnicities due to its premise of honoring clients' context and acknowledgment of multiple realities. In narrative therapy, clients are regarded as the author and expert of their own story, and its non-pathologizing approach may make Chinese individuals feel more comfortable despite the cultural stigma of receiving mental health services (Chen, 2012).

Because Chinese individuals seem particularly receptive to external influences in the mate selection process, and given the cultural pressure to conform to social expectations and others' opinions, addressing the societal norm of women marrying up and men marrying down might be appropriate when conducting therapy with Chinese women for their mate selection struggles. Therapists may consider highlighting the uniqueness of the client's individual experiences in choosing a spouse, and help the client externalize dominant societal narratives that might be constraining (White & Epston, 1990). For example, Chinese women with a high level of education may be concerned about the scarcity of eligible marriage candidates who satisfy dominant societal expectations, and thus might benefit from examining such expectations in therapy.

Therapists may also be well positioned to help Chinese women who may feel worthless due to their struggles in the mate selection process. Namely, the therapist may be able to help these women become more aware of their own strengths and resources, particularly when their strengths are not those most commonly valued in mate selection, such as physical attraction or financial resources. Therapists can assist clients identify and embrace less commonly emphasized mate selection assets, and in so doing, reconstruct clients' self-perceptions of their position in the mate selection market. Because the difficulty experienced during the mate selection process tends to negatively affect Chinese individuals' sense of self-worth, the technique of externalization, in particular, may help a client see their struggle as separate from themselves, creating space for alternative, more constructive narratives (Morgan, Brosi, & Brosi, 2011; Santos, Goncalves, & Matos, 2011).

At the same time, therapists attempting to use narrative therapy techniques in working with Chinese women struggling with mate selection issues should be mindful of the cultural implications of their words and strive to be unassuming. In particular, when requesting clients to elaborate on their experiences incongruent with external expectations, therapists who are not of the client's culture might face less resistance when asking clients to elaborate more, whereas therapists who are of the client's culture may find it more productive to use personal disclosure to prompt the client to elaborate (Chen, 2012).

Directions for Relationship Education

Aside from working directly with Chinese women struggling with mate selection issues, providing preventive services such as relationship education might prove particularly cost-effective and far-reaching. The purpose of such programs is not to impose specific mate selection values on individuals, but to help participants clarify and prioritize their evolving mate selection values and expectations. These interventions can supplement existing skill-based relationship education programs by addressing relationship conflicts rooted in constraining beliefs and expectations regarding mate selection in general.

For instance, although narratives such as women marrying up are culturally enforced, the open endorsement of such criteria carries negative connotations (e. g., "gold digger"). Consequently, many individuals become ensnared in a double bind. On the one hand, societal norms encourage women to marry up, and on the other hand, judgments await those who openly seek to do so. As such, relationship education classes tailored for Chinese women could acknowledge that it is not uncommon for women to desire marrying someone of higher perceived value than themselves on certain criteria, and that men tend to do likewise with respect to other criteria. As a first step, this knowledge may help normalize the negative connotations associated with women wanting to marry up. The group could then discuss the pros and cons of such thinking, while considering the criteria that may concern personality and values rather than simply possessions, potential earning power, or physical appearance.

Discussion of a wide range of mate selection criteria could create more openness and flexibility. For instance, if a young woman is determined to marry up, she may rule out decent marriage candidates who, on the surface, do not seem to be of higher perceived value according to marriage market criteria. It would be worthwhile to discuss other relationship qualities she may not be considering, such as loyalty, character, commitment to an egalitarian relationship, and the degree to which the potential mate's family of origin exhibits these characteristics. Additionally, although mate selection criteria are inherently value-laden, therapists should avoid assuming which criteria are more important for a particular client. For instance, individuals from collectivistic cultures might emphasize a possible mate's family orientation or feel more comfortable with their parents influencing their mate selection than many clients from individualistic cultures.

Furthermore, relationship education may help challenge unrealistic mate selection expectations that hinder individuals' success in mate selection (e.g., Larson, 1992). Because unrealistic expectations may increase individuals' selection time and felt pressure, individuals should be challenged to prioritize their expectations, and to make appropriate compromises. In this regard, a relationship education class can help Chinese women prioritize their mate selection criteria, and adjust their unrealistic expectations and limiting beliefs (Cobb, Larson, & Watson, 2003). Culturally relevant metaphors might be particularly useful in facilitating such discussions (Zhou, Chiu, & Chui, 2017).

Case Study

Li, 35-year-old, is a recently divorced physician with a punishing work schedule. Her ex-husband Wang, 37-year-old, is an affluent business owner. Li and Wang were introduced through a meeting arranged by their parents and now have a 5-year-old son together. Li and Wang's marriage deteriorated because Wang felt that Li was neglecting her wifely duties in favor of her work. Li, on the other hand, felt Wang was unsupportive, self-centered, and emotionally distant. When Li learned Wang's affair with Zhang, a beautiful 21-year-old college senior, she ended the marriage. After the divorce, Wang started formally dating Zhang immediately.

Li's parents, with whom Li is very close, opposed her decision to divorce Wang and suggested that she forgive Wang, dismissing Wang's affair as a "common transgression for men." When Li pursued the divorce despite their disapproval, they overtly and repeatedly expressed their disappointment with her and seemed ashamed by her decision. They also thought that Li was too stubborn and that her desire for emotional intimacy, too idealistic. Concerned that Li's status as a single mother in her mid-30s would make decent marriage prospects a dismal possibility, which would only worsen as she aged, Li's parents urged her to seek a new husband as soon as possible, constantly arranging blind dates and pressuring her to "not be too picky."

Although Li believed the painful experiences of her first marriage could be largely attributed to its hasty start and the fact that she and Wang held vastly different ideas about marriage, Li felt immense guilt and pressure for "failing and worrying" her parents. An attractive woman and a confident professional, Li started to believe, as her parents suggested, that her age and single-mom status would make it extremely difficult for her to secure a husband, unless she compromised on her mate selection standards. She even began doubting her decision to divorce Wang. As pressure from her parents mounted and efforts in finding a suitable spouse were unfruitful, Li grew more depressed and anxious, which in turn negatively affected her work and relationship with her son.

The therapist hypothesized that Li was poorly differentiated from her family of origin and lacked appropriate boundaries with her parents regarding her mate selection choices. The therapist also hypothesized that Li had internalized the negative and desperate perception of herself as a single-mom divorcee in her mid-30s, based on her parents' comments and the dominant societal narrative for Chinese women in her position. This constraining narrative, the therapist proposed, rendered Li powerless and hopeless.

To promote Li's differentiation from her parents, the therapist interviewed Li about her family history and developed a genogram to facilitate discussion about the relationship patterns in her family of origin. Through this process, Li became more aware of her parents' over-involvement in her life, and the negative impact of their well-intentioned interferences. To prepare Li for potential reactions from her parents as she began establishing firmer boundaries, the therapist predicted that Li's parents might be unaccustomed to the new, healthier boundaries, and encouraged her to recognize their reactions as transactional and temporary, which will eventually calm down if she can maintain the boundaries calmly without becoming emotionally reactive. To help Li reduce her emotional reactivity, the therapist used process questions to help Li process and manage her anxiety.

Li struggled with conflicting feelings regarding her parents' interference of her mate selection: feeling, on the one hand, resentful toward her parents for rushing her into her first marriage that ended painfully and urging her to remarry hastily despite her obvious discomfort and emotional struggle, and on the other hand, guilty for failing her parents by dissolving her marriage and burdening them with worries for her future. The therapist validated her feelings, acknowledging both as meaningful parts of her experiences.

The therapist then explored with Li her intense guilt, which seemed to stem from a constraining definition of being a "good daughter," which entails pleasing her parents at all times and being "successful in life," which entails maintaining a marriage. The therapist reframed Li's decision to terminate her first marriage after learning about her husband's affair, as evidence of her personal integrity, courage, and self-respect, all qualities that Li considered important aspects of her self-identity. Through this process, Li externalized the image of herself as a failure and a disappointment and was able to focus on and affirm her many strengths.

Furthermore, the therapist encouraged Li to take more ownership and authority of her mate selection choice, using "I" statements to state her preferences and requirements in a potential spouse and identify qualities important to her, regardless of how these qualities might be valued by her parents and family of origin. Li identified loyal, responsible, and mature as qualities that would be essential for her potential mate to possess, whereas she previously regarded these qualities as secondary to being a provider and having a good family background, the very qualities that Li's parents prioritized for her.

Conclusions and Recommendations

With sincere curiosity for the mate selection experiences of Chinese women and awareness of the prominent cultural and societal barriers relevant to the Chinese context, therapists would be able to help these women navigate the mate selection process and the many challenges in this process more mindfully. As such, the therapist could contribute to helping these clients lay a more solid foundation for their marital relationship.

References

Chen, R. (2012). Narrative therapy for Chinese adults raised as an only child. *Contemporary Family Therapy*, 34, 104–111.

Chen, R. (2016). Mating gradient. In C. L. Shehan (Ed.), *The Wiley Blackwell encyclopedia of family studies*. Hoboken, NJ: Wiley-Blackwell.

Chen, R., & Austin, J. P. (2017). The effect of external influences on mate selection necessity traits: Cross-cultural comparisons of Chinese and American men and women. *Marriage & Family Review*, 53, 246–261.
Cobb, N. P., Larson, J. H., & Watson, W. L. (2003). Development of the attitudes about romance and mate selection scale. *Family Relations*, 52, 222–231.
Dion, K. K., & Dion, K. L. (1993). Individualistic and collectivistic perspective on gender and the cultural context of love and intimacy. *Journal of Social Issues*, 49, 53–59.
England, P., & McClintock, E. A. (2009). The gendered double standard of aging in U.S. marriage markets. *Population and Development Review*, 35, 797–816.
Epstein, N. B., Berger, A. T., Fang, J. J., Messina, L. A., Smith, J. R., Lloyd, T. D., … Liu, Q. X. (2012). Applying Western-developed family therapy models in China. *Journal of Family Psychotherapy*, 23, 217–237.
Greenberg, L. S., Rice, L. N., & Elliott, R. (1993). *Facilitating emotional change: The moment-by-moment process*. New York: Guilford.
Hu, W., Sze, Y. T., Chen, H., & Fang, X. (2015). Actor-partner analyses of the relationship between family-of-origin triangulation and marital satisfaction in Chinese couples. *Journal of Child and Family Studies*, 24, 2135–2146.
Ji, Y. (2015). Between tradition and modernity: "Leftover" women in Shanghai. *Journal of Marriage and Family*, 77, 1057–1073.
Ji, Y., & Yeung, W. J. (2014). Heterogeneity in contemporary Chinese marriage. *Journal of Family Issues*, 35, 1662–1682.
Jones, G. W., & Gubhaju, B. (2009). Factors influencing changes in mean age at first marriage and proportions never marrying in the low-fertility countries of East and Southeast Asia. *Asian Population Studies*, 5, 237–265.
Jung, M. (1999). The application of marital mediation to Chinese American immigrants. *Family Therapy*, 26, 1–12.
Kerr, M. E., & Bowen, M. (1988). *Family evaluation: An approach based on Bowen theory*. New York: W. W. Norton & Company.
Larson, J. H. (1992). "You're my one and only": Premarital counseling for unrealistic beliefs about mate selection. *American Journal of Family Therapy*, 20, 242–253.
McGoldrick, M., Gerson, R., & Shellenberger, S. (1999). *Genograms: Assessment and intervention* (2nd ed.). New York: W. W. Norton & Company.
Miller, R. B., Anderson, S., & Keals, D. K. (2004). Is Bowen theory valid? A review of basic research. *Journal of Marital and Family Therapy*, 30, 453–466.
Minuchin, S., & Fishman, H. C. (1981). *Family therapy techniques*. Cambridge, MA: Harvard University.
Morgan, M. L., Brosi, W. A., & Brosi, M. W. (2011). Restorying older adults' narratives about self and substance abuse. *The American Journal of Family Therapy*, 39, 444–455.
Santos, A., Goncalves, M., & Matos, M. (2011). Innovative moments and poor outcome in narrative therapy. *Counseling and Psychotherapy Research*, 11, 129–139.
Tian, F. F. (2013). Transition to first marriage in reform-era urban China: The persistent effect of education in a period of rapid social change. *Population Research and Policy Review*, 32, 529–552.
To, S. (2013). Understanding Sheng Nu ("leftover women"): The phenomenon of late marriage among Chinese professional women. *Symbolic Interaction*, 36, 1–20.
Toro-Morn, M., & Sprecher, S. (2003). A cross-cultural comparison of mate preferences among university students: The United States vs. the People's Republic of China (PRC). *Journal of Comparative Family Studies*, 34, 151–170.

Trent, K., & South, S. (2011). Too many men? Sex ratios and women's partnering behavior in China. *Social Forces*, 90, 247–267.

Wang, H., & Abbot, D. (2013). Waiting for Mr. Right: The meaning of being a single educated Chinese female over 30 in Beijing and Guangzhou. *Women's Studies International Forum*, 40, 222–229.

White, M., & Epston, D. (1990). *Narrative means to therapeutic ends*. New York: W. W. Norton & Company.

Zhang, S., & Kline, S. L. (2009). Can I make my own decision? A cross-cultural study of perceived social network influence in mate selection. *Journal of Cross-Cultural Psychology*, 40, 3–23.

Zhou, R. D. H., Chiu, M. Y. L., & Chui, W. (2017). Development and validation of the Marital Metaphor Questionnaire (MMQ-10) for Urban Chinese women. *Journal of Marital and Family Therapy*, 43, 65–81.

Additional Resources

Buunk, A. P., Park, J. H., & Duncan, L. A. (2010). Cultural variation in parental influence on mate choice. *Cross-Cultural Research*, 44, 23–40.

Chen, R., Austin, J. P., Miller, J. K., & Piercy, F. P. (2015). Chinese and American individuals' mate selection criteria: Updates, modifications, and extensions. *Journal of Cross-Cultural Psychology*, 46, 101–118.

Huang, K. (2014). Marriage squeeze in China: Past, present, and future. *Journal of Family Issues*, 35, 1642–1661.

Kerr, M. E., & Bowen, M. (1988). *Family evaluation: An approach based on Bowen theory*. New York: W. W. Norton & Company.

Minuchin, S. (1974). *Families and family therapy*. Cambridge, MA: Harvard University.

Mu, Z., & Xie, Y. (2014). Marital age homogamy in China: A reversal of trend in the reform era? *Social Science Research*, 44, 141–157.

11

HELPING JEWISH COUPLES ADDRESS ISSUES OF GENDER ROLE CONFLICT IN MARRIAGE

Ashley Cooper

Introduction

There are many traditions that the Jewish culture embodies. The construct of marriage within the Jewish faith has been challenged due to the postmodern shift of gender role development. As in many cultures, families attempt to model themselves after the families that raised them, and the generations before. Due to the evolving socioeconomic society, gender roles have shifted from traditional household roles to dual incomes, shared responsibilities with child rearing and shared housekeeping, as well as the attempt to keep up with the Jewish faith. Jewish women and men are shown to earn higher education degrees at above average numbers, creating dual-income earning households on average with their socioeconomic non-Jewish neighbors (Fishman, 2015). However, work in continuing Jewish traditions becomes for many families a 'third-shift' of work, where in many cases additional stress is added due to financial costs and unevenly weighted gendered religious responsibilities (Fishman, 2015).

For some, this was not the marriage they imagined they'd spend their lives navigating, and the realization of these changes can have a devastating impact on their matrimonial harmony. Pressure, guilt, resentments, and anxiety often ensue, resulting in spousal separations for those not getting what they bargained for (Berner, 2018). This bares the question, is society stronger than cultural tradition? And can a marriage that was grounded in the assumptions of following familial institutions be saved if that institution is no longer valid? This chapter will explore the challenges for one Jewish couple as they faced the evolution of gender roles, and the desire to hold onto cultural traditions.

A Brief History of "The Chosen Ones"

According to Hebrew University's Professor Sergio Della Pergola, Jewish people make up less than 0.2% of the world's population, with the majority of those who identify as Jewish living in Israel and the United States of America (Dashefsky, 2017). The relevance of this statistic is understood by the emphasis Jewish culture has in tradition, and when considering the people's limited population – the importance of continuing their Jewish values and rituals increases. Today, many people with Jewish heritage can identify family members who were persecuted due to their religious and cultural beliefs and killed during the Holocaust. Jewish families lived in fear as they were forced to flee their homes, attempting to deny their religious affiliation, and were separated from their families as they were placed on trains and sent to concentration camps.

Nazi Germany, under the rule of Adolph Hitler, saw Jewish people as an inferior race, one that was to be exterminated in an attempt to build a master race of Arian people. An estimated 6 million Jews tragically perished between 1941 and 1945, leaving a sense of urgency in keeping the Jewish faith practiced and honored today (Medoff, 2003). Keeping tradition alive has become a central theme within the modern Jewish communities.

Ask ten different people what comes to mind when they think of Jewish faith, and you'll likely get ten different answers. This is because the Jewish culture has a multitude of subgroups or denominations, which may differ dramatically in their approach towards Jewish traditions, laws, and ritual observance. Presently in the United States, there are five main assemblies of Judaism which are identified as Reform, Conservative, Orthodox, Reconstructionist, and Secular.

The Reformed Jewish community can account for approximately 31% of Jewish people in the United States and is often considered the most "liberal" of the denominations. This movement of Judaism is much smaller internationally but has had significant growth in the United States due to its postmodern way of expressing the culture and religion. The Reformed community was created from an attempt to merge Judaism with modern life and blend it with developing concepts in Western thought (My Jewish Learning, 2018). The Reformed movement can be considered quite progressive as it is politically liberal, egalitarian on gender issues, active in interfaith efforts and religiously open-minded, whereby it accepts the patrilineal decent rather than only matrilineal and ordaining women and LGBTQ as rabbis (MJL, 2018). It has underlined the ethical aspects of Jewish tradition over ritual requirements; however in recent decades it has begun to re-embrace some of the religious practices it once dismissed due to its attempts to stay connected to the faith upon which it grew.

The Conservative branch of Judaism began in the 19th century in reaction to what it perceived to be as "radical nature of Reform Judaism" (Caroll, 2018). Conservative Jews felt the principles adopted by Reformed Judaism had tossed out too much of what is crucial to the Jewish religion. Conservative Judaism takes somewhat of a mid-position between Orthodox and Reform groups – many traditions and practices are retained, but some reforms are instituted as well. Conservative Judaism is the second largest form of Judaism in the United States (Caroll, 2018).

Orthodox Jews are those who preserve the strict traditional beliefs and practices of the faith. They stringently observe the Kosher or "kashrut" dietary laws as well as the practices of the sabbath. This community is more often identified by their traditional manner in dressing. Adult males may wear black suits and hats, and sometimes allow the hair in front of their ears to grow into long curls, called "peyos" (Sherpin, 2017). Women sometimes wear bonnets or other head coverings, and dress in modestly long skirts as well as buttoned-up blouses that cover the arms. Orthodox synagogues are gender segregated and follow gender assigned religious rituals, as according to traditional Jewish law.

The Reconstructionist movement challenged the traditional belief that God could literally choose one people over another, and rejected this idea saying that the idea of privileged access to God promoted dangerous assumptions of superiority (Seltzer, 2018). Rabbi Kaplan defined Judaism as a "civilization" and made it an all-embracing way of life that includes languages, literature, food, customs, civil and criminal law, art, music, food – all elements of any civilization but elements that are usually considered secular (MJL, 2018). This evolution in Judaism served to encourage Jews who felt a lack of a connection from traditional religious Jewish practice to become part of the culture.

Secular Jews are those who identify as Jewish culturally but not religiously. This group feels a sense of pride in their culture but does not always practice the religious aspects of the Jewish faith. While the Secular group identify as Jews and have Jewishness as a core part of their identity, they do not always believe in God or practice the Jewish faith. They are non-religious people who identify as Jewish by culture but not necessarily by religion.

Modern Jewish Families and Relationship Expectations

Navigating through a modern-day marriage is no easy task regardless of one's religious or cultural affiliation. Raising a family, keeping a home, earning sufficient income, balancing love, care, and affection are just a few aspects those in modern day marriages attempt to harmonize. Now consider the added pressure of the media which has invaded our TVs, cell phones, computers, and tablets in telling us what it means to be happy and successful. The stressors of having to worry about our looks is just the icing on the cake of misinformation. Images of happy couples on vacation, or images of children ripping open dozens of beautifully wrapped packages under a Christmas tree becomes what many strive to achieve.

In some cases, the modern Conservative Jews strive to be able to provide their children with the highest level of Jewish *and* secular education; to enjoy the prosperity of modern society while retaining Torah values; to take vacations in Maui with Glatt Kosher meals and of course, capturing it all on a smart phone to show the world how easily this was all able to be achieved and balanced, with bright-eyed little Jordan and Sarah in the backdrop.

Many want a relationship rooted in tradition, sometimes with traditional roles, yet connection and a partnership with a spouse is desired, which historically has been shown not to be considered so traditional. During the time of what was known as the Second Wave of Feminism, the entry of women into the workforce did not completely transform gender relationships within families; rather they have created a "stalled revolution" or an "unfinished revolution" (Hochschild, 2012). The continuing gender division of labor such as expectations for a woman to leave the workplace only to return home to second day of work with child rearing *and* upholding Jewish traditions takes a toll on modern families. Hochschild (2012) defined traditional gender ideology to be with heterosexual female partners doing less paid work and taking care of cooking, cleaning, carpooling, and caregiving more than their male partners, especially when men worked long hours in their paid jobs. However, Hochschild also found that when men had more flexibility or women worked longer hours outside of the home, the impression of the spouses was that the childcare and cooking were more assigned to role of the woman than the male partner.

A 2015 study by Fishman interviewed 15 married Jewish couples and took an in-depth look at how these couples chose to navigate family, work, marriage, and Judaism, with the central theme of Judaism being paralleled to "work." Many Jewish men and women in the modern world enter their marriages expecting some sort of negations regarding the management of different roles. Some couples chose to fall back on dated established gender roles in some areas, but navigate new patterns in others (Fishman, 2015). Respondents of the research noted that these new patterns are a "shift" away from tradition, and that another "shift" they face is the implantation of their faith within in the home. The practice of Judaism for more conservative families take time, energy, and money. However, for many of the respondents in this study, they felt Judaism was "necessary work to frame (or set a foundation for their) families."

In an online survey of 59 Jewish women and men, it was found that dual working couples with children require frequent role negotiations within the home. While those couples who allowed themselves to fall back into older conventional roles, showed signs of marital dissatisfaction (Fishman, 2015). Therefore, when couples are seeking guidance in maintaining a happy relationship while balancing children, dual work schedules, tasks within the home, and Judaism; the adoption of negotiation tactics is crucial. While the idea of negotiating roles is favorable, this cannot work without the ability for both partners to be flexible and willing to follow through on agreements. Stress can result if a partner feels he or she is taking on more work than the partner; likewise when one partner feels the other is not living up to their end of the bargain.

Gender and the Jewish Faith

Research on gender in the United States shows that women are more religious than men, primarily in regard to their frequency of religious services attended (Gerson, 2010). Women are also seen to include more of their faith into their personal beliefs and ways of life (Gerson, 2010). It is likely because of this that researchers have also found that women are disproportionately responsible for both unpaid labor in the home, as well as their family's religious expression (Fishman, 2015). Scholars propose several theories to explain gendered differences in religiosity, including risk-related behaviors, gender role socialization and life-course effects. Hartman (2009) explains this phenomenon to be prevalent within the Jewish community because Jewish women's connections to family-based rituals and roles might be stronger in comparison to their labor force participation. Jewish women exhibited stronger Jewish identities, especially in regard to beliefs, public ritual practices, activity in the community and attachment to the Jewish people (Fishman & Parmer, 2008).

Having stronger ties to the Jewish community and faith, bring increased time commitment as well as financial strain. Maintaining Kashrut often is an added financial expense when compared non-Jewish family's abilities to purchase their weekly meals at lower priced markets than ones that strictly adhere to the laws of Kashrut (or Kosher). In addition to the financial burden, preparation of these meals is time consuming and take a serious level of discipline to maintain within the household for family's that have children. This time constraint may impede the ability to work of the one who does the purchases and prepares the food, completes other household chores, and it causes increased levels of stress. Often, the management of the family's ability to maintain Kashrut in modern days has diminished with more dual working households, which again causes stress and feelings of guilt among those in the Jewish faith.

Case Study

"Aaron," age 33, and "Sylvia," age 31, decided to seek couples counseling after a series of arguments they had been having over a period of just under one year, led them to feel "hopeless," and "perhaps just too different to last." The couple had been married for six years and had two daughters together ages 2 and 5. Aaron and Sylvia identify as Jewish; however, Aaron identified as Conservative and Sylvia identified as "more Reformed," and somewhat "Secular." Though Aaron knew Sylvia was not "as religious" as him before they were married, the couple did not feel this would cause an issue in their life together as they reported being "head over heels" for each other and felt they could make anything work. The couple's families got along well with one another, and Sylvia reported that their fathers "grew up together" in the late 1950s in a small Jewish neighborhood, which made their bond feel that much more significant as they had strong family and community connections.

Prior to getting married, Aaron had completed law school and was starting out as a young lawyer in a prominent law firm in their town. Sylvia worked in a school for children with special needs, and after the birth of their first child, she returned to school to obtain her master's degree in social work. Shortly after the completion of her course work in her school program, she found out she was pregnant with their second child. Due to complications during her pregnancy, she was unable to complete the internship portion of her program and was forced to take time off school. Sylvia recalls being "devastated" in having to put her program on hold, but ultimately knew it was the best thing for their unborn child. After their second daughter was born healthy, Sylvia wanted to return to complete her program, but Aaron had decided it would cost too much money to put both children in a "suitable" Jewish preschool and daycare and told Sylvia she needed to stay home until both girls were ready to go to school full time. Sylvia tried convincing Aaron that there were other programs for their daughters that were much less costly; however, they were not Jewish programs, and Aaron declined.

Aaron reported "trying to understand" Sylvia wanting to go back to school, to finish what she started, and suggested she volunteer at their synagogue a few days a week where they had programs for children. Sylvia decided some time out of the house would be good for her, and the girls could stay with her sister who was a stay-at-home mother during those few hours. Sylvia disclosed that she "hated" working at the synagogue and felt judged for not being "as Jewish" as many of the other women who worked there. Sylvia did not remember much of the Hebrew she learned as a child and did not feel passionate about services, or "high holidays." Sylvia recalls a group of women "jokingly" pointing out that Sylvia would never host holidays because she "did not know how to prepare Kashrut." Aaron had been raised Kosher in his home, while Sylvia had not. Aaron disclosed that he felt "let down" due to Sylvia saying she would learn how to prepare meals according to Jewish law so that he could continue his traditions, but she had not made an attempt to do so. Aaron also stated upon getting married the couple had agreed to have three children and he was eager to complete their family. Sylvia grew up alongside one other sibling, while Aaron had six brothers and sisters, and always wanted a big family of his own. In fact, Aaron felt he was compromising in having only three children. Sylvia said she would not consider having another child until she was able to finish her master's degree and begin working as a social worker so that she could contribute to the family's finances and have her own career.

Sylvia stated she felt that Aaron did not understand her frustration with having to "conform" to his ways of Judaism and that he was being selfish. She disagreed with his previous statement, and affirms she did try to cook Kosher for the family but between household work, volunteering, and taking care of two young children, she was frustrated with the time it took to prepare, and was uncomfortable with how expensive it was when considering the money, she felt they could save by secular eating. Though Sylvia was Jewish she reported feeling "never Jewish enough" and agitated with other women at their synagogue who would make jokes, sometimes to Aaron about Sylvia's non-commitment to the community. Finally, the couple's oldest daughter had started kindergarten at a Hebrew school for Conservative Jewish children, and Sylvia was concerned with the costs, her inability to help her daughter with her Hebrew homework, and feelings of being "different" from the other mothers in the classroom which made organizing play dates for their daughter challenging. Furthermore, Sylvia's concerns over finances, her inability to complete her degree and begin work to assist in earning income, added stress over the prospect of having a third child. Meanwhile, Aaron reported feeling "deceived" and "disappointed," that his wife appeared to have reneged on their agreement to have three children and to raise the family closer to the Conservative way of Jewish life.

Case Study

When considering the case of Aaron and Sylvia, there is a pyramid of emotional breakdown that has occurred with a central theme rooted in the decline of their relationship. While it would appear the central issue regarding their arguments is religion, this would be ignoring the origin of where their communication was deteriorating. Expectations are the central theme that have become the root upon where, criticism, defensiveness, stonewalling, and contempt have begun to grow. According to Gottman's studies, the "four horsemen" aforementioned can be predictors of divorce (Gottman, 2007): "contempt," "stonewalling," "defensiveness," and "criticisim."

Couples who function in a healthy manner often treat each other with consideration and are supportive of each other. Without these basic characteristics, relationships often become muddled with resentments and lingering arguments. A central goal in treating Aaron and Sylvia was increasing their intimacy as well as friendship behaviors, addressing conflict productively and timely, and building a life together with a shared meaning. Considering the root of their arguing was expectations due to their differences in how they chose to practice Judaism, this would not be an easy task. It would be necessary for the couple to learn to compromise and stick to their agreements, while understanding and empathizing with each other's chosen way of life and spirituality.

Aaron and Sylvia both reported feeling a hurried need for marriage counseling in order to save their relationship and to keep their homelife stable. Sylvia repeatedly said she loved her husband Aaron, but felt unhappy with how things were going, and wanted to work on finding a way to love each other as they once did. Aaron also stated he loved his wife and felt stuck and frustrated with her unhappiness. Both felt working on their marriage was exceedingly important since they had children and were willing to fight to keep their family together. Having two committed persons who appear to be truthful in loving each other and wanting to work on their issues makes the process of marriage counseling have a higher chance of success (Gottman, 2007). Their commitment to their family served as a strength in treatment. On the other end of the spectrum, Aaron and Sylvia had very different ideas of how to express their religious beliefs and how they feel they should include Judaism within their children's lives. Furthermore, Aaron was eager to have another child and Sylvia was eager to go back to school and regain some of her independence. Both persons have catastrophized their differences and allowed these challenges to create a void in their vision of what they want for their family.

An eclectic mix of narrative therapy and Gottman's principles were utilized to work with this couple. "Narrative therapy is a method that separates the person(s) from the problem and encourages people to rely on their own skill sets to minimize the problems that exist in their everyday lives" (Morgan, 2000). Narrative therapy is beneficial to couples as it is non-pathologizing and aims to empower while creating a collaboration between the couple and their therapist. Aaron and Sylvia's unique competencies, skills, and expertise were used to serve as a catalyst to promote change within their life together. It was important to view both partners as separate from their problems which promoted success in externalizing sensitive issues such as how to express their religion, and differences on when to potentially have another child. In order to empower Aaron and Sylvia's relationship, the goal was not to transform either of them, rather to transform the negative impacts their issues have had on their relationship. The objective was to distance the couple from their identified problems in an attempt to make it possible to see how their differences may be serving them, rather than harming them.

Creating the Narrative

After the couple's initial session, where they both expressed their dedication to the process of counseling and in saving their marriage, as well as identifying their perceived marital issues, they attended a second session one week later. Each person had been tasked with "creating their narrative," a process upon which they tell their story in their own words (Standish, 2013). This process was utilized in order help the couple develop their unique and individual stories to give them an opportunity to discover meaning and assist each other in better understanding the "why" to what they hold onto as important such as religion, work, and family. In this case, this technique was also used to "re-author" as the clients explored their own experiences to find alterations to their story in order to release them from being anchored to ideals that were negatively impacting their current marriage and future family dynamic.

The couple's narrative creation process took three one-hour sessions, with homework included. Sylvia insisted that Aaron share first, therefore the first session was dedicated to the discovery of Aaron's story which included his childhood and family life, with memories of his mother that were very present in his narrative. The themes of love, Judaism, food and sibling closeness were woven together seamlessly, and successfully painted a clear picture as to why Aaron felt so strongly about Kosher meals, and a large family with his wife Sylvia at the center of it all.

Sylvia found this process to be more challenging than Aaron had, and she stated she wasn't sure how to make her narrative "meaningful." Sylvia admitted she struggled with this assignment more so after she heard her husband share his. "His story made so much sense, it tied everything together and it was so clear why he cares so much that we raise our family in a similar way to how he was raised," Sylvia said. She expressed that she felt her story was "vague," and she struggled to find any reasons for why she valued work and independence so much. However, upon sharing her narrative it became evident not just to Aaron but to Sylvia as well why she did not desire a big family and why she struggled with the demands of keeping a Kashrut home. Sylvia's family was more Secular than Aarons, and she was mostly able to eat what she wanted. Judaism was important but primarily on the "high holidays." Furthermore, Sylvia's sister whom she reported to looking up to, loosely converted to Buddhism and married a man who shared her spirituality. The couple had no children and traveled frequently, sharing their experiences and unique gifts with their family when they returned home, sparking a twinge of jealousy in Sylvia. Sylvia soon realized that she longed for some sense of something to "call (her) own." Therefore, her ability to work and establish herself in a career was important.

An interesting and fun thing about the clinical process is the unintentional threadwork that appears with different styles and modalities. By Aaron and Sylvia successfully putting together their narratives, they were able to include a very useful 'Deconstruction Technique.' "Deconstruction" refers to breaking down the problem or problems the client(s) are having, making it easier to understand and address. While problems can often feel overwhelming, agitating, or unsolvable, they never truly are if the people involved are dedicated to solving them (Bishop, 2011). Deconstructing the issues in this case through narrative story-telling, made the couple's problems more specific and clarified what the core issues were. In this case, the deconstruction technique was utilized quite unintentionally with Aaron and Sylvia, who were having trouble in their marriage. Aaron was feeling frustrated with Sylvia who to him, appeared to not value his family goals. Sylvia was hurt by Aaron who seemed to not value her growth in a different direction, and desire to be happy by fostering a sense of independence. While this was part of the basis of the couple's issue, they were able to use their narrative story-telling to break down those matters while discovering what each problem meant to them on a much deeper level. This method again acted as a catalyst to understanding and empowerment in assisting the couple in finding a solution. Deconstructing the problem helped the couple to learn *exactly* what the problem was and why it was so important to each person, which created a sense of empathy between Aaron and Sylvia.

After the Why, Comes the How

Now that Aaron and Sylvia had uncovered why they were each having such strong emotions regarding their positions, they needed to figure out how they were going to work past their issues. Deep seeded issues do not change overnight, and it was not likely that Aaron and Sylvia were going to change how they felt about their desired way of life. However, arming the couple with understanding became the foundation upon which a tower of compromise was constructed. Just as problems have roots, solutions have foundations where basic needs in a relationship can be built.

Aaron and Sylvia were four sessions into their therapy when they began working towards creating a solution. While this may sound like a quick process, remember, it is easy to identify a problem and come up with a solution, but maintaining that solution is where the real work begins. Each person was tasked with identifying areas they felt they could compromise on, and areas they absolutely could not compromise on, no matter the outcome. This was an important step to take as religious beliefs and the will to bear children are deeply personal choices that if altered unwillingly can lead to unrepairable resentments. In this case, Sylvia was open to having another child, and was able to be flexible on this issue; her compromise in this case was to complete school first and get a solid footing in the workforce. This would give both Aaron and Sylvia their way as he would see their family grow and Sylvia would feel more able to contribute financially and more comfortable with another child added to the mix. Furthermore, she would have a career that was hers aside from motherhood and Judaism.

Regarding Judaism, this was a more challenging area as Aaron was not as willing to budge on his beliefs in keeping the house Kashrut. This struggle took the clients into their sixth session where Sylvia came armed with financials. She was able to show Aaron how much more expensive their Kosher diets would be per month in comparison to keeping a "loose" Kosher diet. Once Aaron saw the numbers, it appeared the couple were finally on the same page and were able to come to an agreement. Until Sylvia was working at least part time, they would keep Kosher part time, or for the Jewish High Holidays. This satisfied Aaron's personal worship goals while also being quite happy about saving some money; after all they were planning to add another member to the family.

Aaron and Sylvia were a typical case with a not so typical outcome. In today's society, religion, gender roles, and economics have become exceedingly challenging to navigate within the realm of marriage. Those who wish to remain rooted in more traditional views may have a difficult time if one partner prefers modernism. Economic factors force couples to take inventory of what they find to be the most important aspects in their homes and to look at what they can and cannot do without. Couples who are armed with the willingness to compromise and utilize maintenance techniques such as check-in and counseling may have better odds of making it through periods of marital adjustment and growth.

Aaron and Sylvia remained in counseling for seven months, and finalized their treatment when Sylvia began the final portion of her social work degree, due to time constraints. The couple last reported doing well and are actively working together in maintaining their compromises with the understanding that different phases in life will bring necessary adjustment.

References

Berner, A. (2018). Modern Orthodox, modern marriages and modern divorces. Jewish Link. Retrieved from www.jewishlinknj.com/monthly-sections/family-link/23898-modern-orthodox-modern-marriages-and-modern-divorces.

Bishop, W. H. (2011). Narrative therapy summary. Retrieved from www.thoughtsfromatherapist.com/2011/05/16/narrative-therapy-summary/.

Caroll, B. (2018). Orthodox Jews, and Reform, Conservative & Secular Jews. World Religions Professor. Retrieved from www.world-religions-professor.com/orthodox-jews.html.

Dashefsky, A., & Sheskin, I. (2017). Jewish population in the United States, 2017. In *American Jewish Year Book* (pp. 202–203). Dordrecht: Springer.

Fishman, B. (2015). *Love, marriage and Jewish families*. Lebanon, NH: Brandeis University Press.

Fishman, B., & Parmer, D. (2008). *Matrilineal ascent/ patrilineal descent: The gender imbalance in American Jewish life*. Waltham, MA: Center for Modern Jewish Studies.

Gerson, K. (2010). *The unfinished revolution: Coming of age in a new era of gender, work, and family*. New York: Oxford University Press.

Gottman, J. (2007). *And a baby makes three*. New York: Three Rivers Press.

Hartman, H., & Hartman, M. (2009). *Gender and American Jews: Patterns in work, education, and family in contemporary life*. Lebanon, NH: Brandeis University Press.

Hochschild, A. (2012). *The second shift: Working families and the Revolution at home*. London: Penguin Books.

Medoff, R. (2003). France and war criminals. *National Review*. Retrieved from www.nationalreview.com/2003/05/france-war-criminals-rafael-medoff/.

Morgan, A. (2000). *What is narrative therapy? An easy to read introduction*. Adelaide: Dulwich Centre Publications.

My Jewish Learning. (2018). History of the Reform movement: America's largest Jewish denomination, Reform began in 19th-century Germany. My Jewish Learning. Retrieved from www.myjewishlearning.com/article/reform-judaism/.

Seltzer, R. (2018). *Mordecai Kaplan: Founder of Reconstructionist Judaism: An examination of the philosophy of one of the 20th century's most prominent Jewish thinkers*. My Jewish Learning. Retrieved from www.myjewishlearning.com/article/mordecai-kaplan-founder-of-reconstructionist-judaism/.

Sherpin, Y. (2017). Jewish identity. Chabad Learning and Values. Retrieved from www.chabad.org/library/article_cdo/aid/42624/jewish/Jewish-Identity.htm.

Standish, K. (2013). Introduction to narrative therapy. Retrieved from https://positivepsychologyprogram.com/narrative-therapy/.

Additional Resources

Gottman, J., & Gottman. J. (2007). *10 lessons to transform your marriage*. New York: Random House.

12

MARRIAGE AND FAMILY COUNSELING IN SAUDI ARABIA

Abeer Ali Rasheed and Mehmet Nurullah Akkurt

Introduction

Please write down three things you believe you know about Saudi Arabia. This will give you an opportunity to evaluate the accuracy of your assumptions as you read about Saudi culture throughout this chapter. We encourage you to reflect upon what you write down as you read this chapter.

Dimensions of Saudi Culture

Individualism and collectivism are the two cultural dimensions used to analyze individuals' social systems, morality, religion, cognitive differentiation, cultural patterns, values, and the embedded self versus the autonomous self (Triandis, 1993). Different than the case in the individualist society, in the collectivist societies, social behavior is predicted from norms, obligations, and responsibilities, and relationships are considered to have the greatest importance for individuals, even if these relationships interfere with personal benefits (Rasheed, 2015). It is important to note that in some cultures people may fall along a continuum, as they are not completely individualist or collectivist. The Saudi culture used to be purely collectivist; however, in the recent years, the new generation in the Saudi society can be described as close to collectivist, but not purely collectivist, which means that those individuals start to depend more on themselves with little boundaries of their own. This slight shift is causing a disturbance in the relations across generations, as more and more youth in Saudi Arabia have started to present certain individualistic values and behaviors.

The current shift of individualistic behavior of the young generation influenced the gender roles as well. Saudi culture is categorized as masculine, in which men are perceived as dominant, strong, and the bread-winner. Women, on the other hand, are perceived as sensitive emotional and they are given the roles of rearing children and taking care of household chores (Brinson & Al-Amri, 2005). However, these roles are also changing in which women nowadays can contribute more in the society and share financial responsibilities with men. Despite clear progress of the women's role the Saudi society, old generations are still against accepting these new roles assumed by the young women in Saudi Arabia.

Along with a predominantly collectivist worldview, Saudi culture tends to be of high context rather than of a low context such as in the American society. Communication in high context cultures is less direct, formal, and information is roundabout and implicit. This type of communication is very sensitive to non-verbal messages such as voice tone, eye movement, and facial expression. The human relationships and the feelings of others are highly considered in high-context communication (Klyukanov, 2005). Saudi individuals are not verbal when it comes to communicating their feelings; they would rather give non-verbal clues, which is expected to be understood by the person on the other end of the communication.

Current Status on Mental Health in Saudi Arabia

According to World Health Organization's Mental Health Atlas (2014), Saudi Arabia has an available stand-alone Mental Health Policy and Mental Health Legislation, of which the former is partially implemented and the latter is not implemented. Total reported mental health inpatient care staff were 4,837. Considering Saudi Arabia's total population (29,369,427), there are only 16.5 mental health professionals per 100,000. There are 24 mental health facilities in the kingdom (inpatient and outpatient), and only 4 general hospitals have psychiatric units. It was reported that, per 100,000 population, there were only 2.13 psychiatrists and 1.38 psychologists.

The report also included that there is an existing Family Program what is focused on parental/family mental health. Although the above numbers are promising for a developing country, there must be an examination of the quality of the training and services of these professionals. The Ministry of Health in Saudi Arabia prepared an update (2015) to WHO Mental Health Atlas, which provided more details regarding the current status of mental health services. Authors discussed that, in Saudi Arabia, many mental health workers' education and qualifications may not be in accordance with the concrete definition provided by WHO (Al-Habeeb, Helmi, & Qureshi, 2016). They further reported that mental health professionals assigned to provide services may not have the necessary clinical experience or the post-graduate degrees as required in developed countries. Authors recommended that this gap could be filled with in-service training programs.

The Saudi Family System

Saudi Arabia is a conservative Muslim country, and Islam is the cultural, religious, and political system. The country derives its legislation from Islam. The rules applied in the country are taken from the Holy book of Quran and the sayings (Hadith) of prophet Mohammad, peace be upon him. The country is fundamentally based on strong religious values, and beliefs. The Islamic beliefs and values shape individuals' life style, attitude, norms, values, roles, and authority.

The family is considered a fundamental core in the Saudi culture. The family system is very solid and the relationship between family members is built upon respect. People rely on family connection for safety, support, power, and well-being. It is a hierarchical system, with regard to age and gender. The elders in the family are expected to be admired by the younger members. Males are expected to be respected in the family and they are given a special responsibility toward their wives and children. Despite a clear change in the role of the women in the family and the community, their main responsibility is rearing children.

Different from the Western concept of marriage, in the Eastern culture in general and in Saudi Arabia specifically marriage is considered a family affair, in which a partner is chosen by the family with respect to the opinion of the son or daughter. In Saudi culture, it is common for partners to get to know each other more after the marriage. Marriage gives status to the individual in the society, and it is seen as a sign of maturity. Married women have more freedom and fewer restrictions from parents compared to single women. Although divorce is an option in the Saudi legal system, it is seen as the last reserve because the idea of divorce is not culturally accepted. Thus, divorced women in Arab societies can suffer emotionally, and have poor prospects, such as being the second wife of a married man (Al-Krenawi, Graham, Dean, & Eltaiba, 2004).

As mentioned, the family system is a unique and closed unit and members are expected to support each other. This support includes dealing with members' conflicts, concerns, and psychological needs. People in the Middle East in general are against disclosing family affairs and individual concerns out of the family system (Brinson & Al-Amri, 2005). In the Saudi culture in specific, family issues is considered to be private, and it is not appropriate to be disclosed out of the nuclear family system. The family as a unit is responsible to deal with the marriage issues in discretion when they occur. It is not to be shared even with the extended family system unless necessary. Elderly members are preserved as the wise who have a long life experience, and they are expected to play the "all knowing" role in the family. When it comes to a mental health issues, which is seen as a stigma that prevent many individuals from seeking help in the Middle East in general (Sewilam et al., 2015), it is considered to be a sign of weakness and shame. Thus, the responsibility of dealing with such case is automatically given to the elder members in the family. Even though seeking help from an elderly family member can be a great asset, it could also be troubling as the elder member is not immune to stigma associated with mental health and can blame the family member seeking help with being weak. All these aspects combined complicate the role of marriage and family counselor in Saudi Arabia.

Therapeutic Interventions When Working with Saudi Families and Couples

Therapists have been using two main approaches when working with culturally diverse families: a culture-specific model and a universal-perspective model. Although the common practice is toward culture-specific approaches, both models have pros and cons. The universal-perspective model is criticized for being too generic, while the culture-specific model is associated with stereotyping of diverse groups. Although the culture-specific model does stereotype culturally diverse groups, as it provides common characteristics of the respective cultures in an organized manner, the key is the clinical judgment of the practitioner to be mindful of the fact the within group differences can be greater than between group differences. Dwairy (2006) was inspired by two main biases (alpha and beta) introduced by Hare-Mustin and Marecek in respect to gender, and he applied these to culture. He argued that alpha bias would mean to exaggerate the differences between the cultures, while beta bias would be denying the differences that exist between cultures. Dwairy (2006) in his book *Counseling and Psychotherapy with Arabs and Muslims* discusses in detail how Western theories are reductionist and unidimensional, and how "it does not fit the holistic personality of Arabs, for whom the individual is an inseparable part of the family and for whom thoughts, emotions, values, and body are one undivided entity" (p. 49).

One of the biggest challenges a Western therapist might face is understanding that when a client belonging to a collectivist culture, such as a Saudi client, walks into the session, it is not solely the individual that counselors needs to work with but all the systems which surround that individual. Al-Krenawi and Graham (2005) asserted that counselors must be sensitive to the fact that culture plays an active co-participant role in treatment when working with Arabs and Muslims. To accomplish that, counselors must have a frame of reference and understanding of what works better with these clients. Solution-Focused Brief Therapy (SFBT) is commonly used when working with Arab or Asian clients, simply due to the fact that both cultures present highly collectivist values. SFBT fits with the therapeutic expectations of an Arab client because of the following:

- It requires minimal disclosure, and focuses more on thoughts.
- It is solution-focused.
- It is strengths-based.
- It is short-term.

- It asks questions regarding the exceptions when the issue was not present. This allows clients to find strength and possible solutions to their issues.
- It utilized the Miracle Question, which allows clients to imagine what their life would look like when the issue is resolved.

Techniques utilized in SFBT, in general, are culture free, and they can be utilized with various clientele. However, when utilizing the Miracle Question, therapists are invited to consider the appropriateness, as this question may suggest that there is a supernatural phenomenon, which is against Islamic belief. Counselors can gather a great deal of information toward solutions from clients' responses to this particular question. When working with Arabs, we urge counselors to refrain from using the word "miracle" as this can cause discomfort for the client. You will find how this question can be appropriately utilized with an Arab client at the end of the chapter when reading the session script between the counselor and Sara.

Finally, although we highly recommend that counselors may use SFBT as an option when working with Saudi clients, there are other approaches, such as CBT, that have been found to work effectively with this population. The key is in choosing an approach that focuses more on thoughts, requires minimal self-disclosure, is goal-oriented, and accounts for the system which the client belongs to. Al-Krenawi and Graham (2000) stated that when working with Arabs, there should be an "emphasis on short-term, directive treatment; communication patterns that are passive and informal; patients' understanding of external loci of control and their use of ethno-specific idioms of distress; and, where appropriate, the integration of modern and traditional healing systems" (p. 9).

Case Example

Sara is 32-year-old female who has been married for ten years. She has four children. After finishing her bachelor's degree in public health, she started working in a government hospital. After long consideration, she decided to seek counseling. Sara explained to her counselor that she has been facing conflict with her husband regarding her work. Her husband is not happy with her working in a male–female mixed environment. On top of the intensive responsibility she has in and outside home, her husband is not willing to assist her in the house. When she asks for help, the husband quotes "Your home is your main responsibility, if you need help, you need it at work." Even though she is contributing to house budget, it is not appreciated. Half-way into the session, the counselor explained that it might be feasible for her husband to be included via phone call, should he accept it. However, Sara was hesitant to share with her husband that she is seeing a professional counselor for help.

Below is an abridged transcription from the first session with Sara:

COUNSELOR: You mentioned earlier that it was not an easy decision for you to seek counseling. What made you come today?

SARA: I was about to quit my job because it is better for my family. So I decided to see a counselor before quitting because it is not what I really want to do.

COUNSELOR: What do you really want to do?

SARA: I want to keep my job, but also be appreciated and supported at home. The world is changing but my husband seems to use the old tradition in his advantage.

COUNSELOR: What do you mean by that?

SARA: He believes all the house chores and taking care of children is wife's responsibility, and the husband is responsible for making money for the family.

COUNSELOR: Have you ever spoken about this concern with friends and family?

SARA: Yes, my mom seem to agree with my husband that she thinks my main role is at home, but at the same time she does not want me to quit my job, but she does not approve for me to be working in a male–female mixed environment. My friends seem to agree with me though.

COUNSELOR: I am glad to hear that you have been seeking help first from friends and family, and now from a professional. This is indication that you really want to find a solution.

SARA: Yes, I do. I want to be able to keep my job and not feel guilty about it.

COUNSELOR: What do you think would be helpful for us to do in our time together to help you find what you are looking for?

SARA: I think my husband needs to be here with me, because he is in the center of the issue.

COUNSELOR: I think that would be good idea; however, as a female counselor, I would not be able to provide services to a man. Currently, only medical doctors and psychiatrists have that privilege. However, we can ask him to join the session via phone conference. What do you think about that?

SARA: Well, I am not sure about if he would be willing to join and even talk about this. I do not have much power over him. I can bring it up and to see what he would say.

COUNSELOR: I must say your willingness to work toward a solution is strength of yours. You are open and willing to try everything. Now, can you please think of a time where this was not an issue.

SARA: Thank you. It was an issue since the beginning; however, I told him that I would only marry him if he allowed me to work when our parents first introduced us. He seemed to agree then. However, it became more difficult to manage after having children and getting promoted at work. I have more responsibilities at work and at home now.

COUNSELOR: It has been rough for you lately, what have you been doing to take care of yourself?

SARA: I have been praying a lot about it. My faith has been my biggest strength. Also, I have a great support from my friends.

COUNSELOR: This is great. I want you to keep doing that to take care of yourself. Now, going back to including your husband in the session, if it is ok with you, I would like us to meet for couple of sessions until we have a better sense of the issue, before including your husband. Is that ok with you?

SARA: Yes, I think this is good idea.

COUNSELOR: Alright. Now, until next session, I want to give you homework. I want you to imagine that you woke up one day and realize this issue you are facing is gone. I want you to write down how is your life different now that this issue is gone. You can be as detailed as you wish.Now let's break down what counselor did with the Sara with consideration of contextual issues.

(We urge you write down what you observed in this communication before further reading.)

- The Family Counselor kept the conversation focused on Sara's thoughts instead of her emotions. This is an important aspect to remember when working with Saudis or Arabs in general that self-disclosure is not easy for individuals raised in a collectivist and high-context culture. Asking clients to share their feelings in the earlier sessions could cause them to withdraw. Therefore counselors must focus on thoughts and cognitive processes until the rapport is built.
- Counselor adhered to a strength-based approach which has been found to work more effectively with Arab clients. Focusing on strengths provides encouragement for the clients, who have already made the hard decision to seek help from an outsider. There is a stigma associated with receiving help, except for medical reasons, from an outsider in collectivist culture. It can be seen as a betrayal of one's community. Therefore, counselors must be mindful of the fact that a client seeking counseling despite the communal pressure deserves to be validated for his or her action.
- Arab clients would want to find a practical solution to their issues with minimal self-disclosure. Therefore, Sara's counselor did not ask her questions that will require Sara to share detailed information, which may be an option for later session after the rapport is built.
- Counselor asked Sara if she had any support from the people around her. This is a strength found in collectivist societies. One of the reasons individuals in collectivist societies do not seek counseling is due to fact that they often find the needed support in their community. Counselor must recognize this strength and encourage client to utilize this resource. Clients can find comfort talking to people that they already know and trust in their communities, without feeling the guilt of betrayal of talking to an outsider.

- We would like to remind that this information should allow you to have a frame of reference when working with a Saudi client; however, you must be conscious of alpha and beta biases explained earlier in this chapter.
- There were certain clues given by Sara that would play a significant role in understanding the issue, but the counselor chose to not discuss in this session, such as gender roles, power difference between husband and wife, generational differences between mothers and daughters, arranged marriage, religion, and faith. A counselor without any background knowledge on Arabic and Islamic culture might want to explore these issues right on spot to inform himself or herself. In most cases, it is professional conduct of a counselor to ask clarifying questions when there is a cultural difference; however, counselors must be conscious that the clarifying questions are asked because it would contribute to the session, not to satisfy counselors' curiosity. There could be a case where a counselor is not well-informed regarding some of the contextual issues that are specific to Saudi or Arab culture. In this case, counselor can hold onto some questions for the next session and do the research later, rather than distracting clients with clarification questions which may not contribute to the session at the time.

Finally, it is a family counselor's ethical and professional responsibility to be aware of their biases, and not impose their values on clients. A Western counselor, who is raised in an individualistic society, might unintentionally blame Sara for giving more power to her husband or for being married in an arranged setting, forgetting the most fundamental fact about Arab cultures. Counselors working with a client who has a different background from theirs must be reflective of their work and examine the potential biases within and outside the session.

Challenges When Working with Saudi Families and Couples

Dealing with Saudi families can be a challenge for Saudi as well as non-Saudi counselors as many factors related to cultural context of Saudi Arabia interfere with the therapeutic process. First of all, the challenge that faces the Saudi counselors can be related to the fact that Saudi Arabia has a gender-segregated society. Males and females are separated from the age of 7, and from that age they do not have a direct communication with each other. Being raised in this environment might impact the work of the counselors with couples as one of the spouses might resist communicating with a counselor of an opposite gender. Saudi society is male-dominant and gender differences are strong (Al-Krenawi & Graham, 2000). Thus, female counselors might struggle while dealing with couples or with a male client as he might not trust her ability simply because of gender. Moreover, in Saudi society, individuals' beliefs and values are rooted in the teaching of Islam, which can be a challenge for professional counselors who use modern psychological methods to reach the potential of those clients (Brinson & Al-Amri, 2005).

Non-Saudi counselors must also consider the mistrust of Saudi clients due to cultural gap. In the Saudi culture, individuals learned that sharing private issues is usually done within the nuclear family system. Thus, trusting an outsider, who is from different culture, is not an easy step to take. Disclosure of personal issues, especially marital concern, is a challenge for both counselors and their clients.

Another important aspect for counselors to know and be prepared for is that they might be dealing with a multi-spousal/multi-parental family. As Saudi law allows polygamy, it is not uncommon to for a counselor to encounter a Saudi man with multiple wives. This is a challenge for all counselors, whether domestic or foreign, working in Saudi Arabia. Such families are likely to experience conflict and hostility between spouses and siblings. When working with such families, counselors may work toward improvement of communication between family members and reducing intra-subfamily hostility (Al-Krenawi, 1998).

Conclusions and Recommendations

The fields of counseling, psychology, and family therapy are given more attention in the Kingdom of Saudi Arabia. Saudi individuals nowadays realize the importance of these fields in their lives with the presence of recent factors that trigger the need for mental health interventions in the Saudi society. Some of these factors are associated with the change of the lifestyle of the society, specifically youth, as discussed earlier. The other factors are associated with the fact that the Middle East in general and Saudi Arabia in specific are facing a violent political conflict. The high rates of war in the area resulting from the current political crisis are causing severe trauma issues not only for individuals and families who are experiencing them but also for those who witness it. Also, the presence of terrorism in the area is causing a major stress for families, as parents are overwhelmed to protect their youth from extremist ideology in such an environment. Individuals and families in Saudi Arabia need an urgent intervention that can deal successfully with their needs and concerns.

As the country currently relies on mental health professionals recruited from neighboring countries, there is an urgent need for Saudi universities to provide training programs in the mental health fields for Saudi nationals. Although some Saudi universities provide either a diploma or master of arts degree in counseling (Brinson & Al-Amri, 2005), there is limited emphasis given to clinical training due to lack of sites for students to complete internships. Moreover, the Saudi government has taken the initiative to send students abroad with full scholarship to study in the hard and social science field, so they may be trained and return back to country. These students play a crucial role in the development of the country once they return, especially in the social fields as they challenge the stigma.

Since Saudi Arabia relies mostly on mental health professionals from other countries, there must be a multicultural training of these counselors prior to their work with Saudi clients. To work professionally and ethically with Saudi families, counselors are encouraged to give special attention to understanding the relationships and roles of individuals within the family (Dwairy, 2006).

Based on the above overview of the Saudi culture, clinical recommendations for working with families from Saudi Arabia include:

- Being aware of the Saudi cultural context and the family system.
- Being aware of the role of the family members, depending on the gender and age.
- Being aware the fundamental Islamic values and beliefs that shape the individual's life style.
- Being aware of the slight movement of the new generation toward being more individualistic.
- Being sensitive to the stigma associated with mental health in Saudi society.
- Being sensitive toward the issue of privacy in the Saudi society.

References

Al-Habeeb, A., Helmi, B., & Qureshi, N. (2016). Mental and social health atlas: An update, Ministry of Health, Saudi Arabia, 2015. *International Neuropsychiatric Disease Journal*, 6(3), 1–20.

Al-Habeeb, A. A., & Qureshi, N. A. (2010). Mental and social health atlas I in Saudi Arabia: 2007–2008 [Atlas 2007–2008 de la santé mentale et sociale en Arabie Saoudite]. *Eastern Mediterranean Health Journal*, 16(5), 570.

Al-Krenawi, A. (1998). Family therapy with a multiparental/multispousal family. *Family Process*, 37(1), 65–81.

Al-Krenawi, A., & Graham, J. R. (2000). Culturally sensitive social work practice with Arab clients in mental health settings. *Health & Social Work*, 25(1), 9–22.

Al-Krenawi, A., & Graham, J. R. (2005). Marital therapy for Arab Muslim Palestinian couples in the context of reacculturation. *The Family Journal*, 13(3), 300–310.

Al-Krenawi, A., Graham, J. R., Dean, Y. Z., & Eltaiba, N. (2004). Cross-national study of attitudes towards seeking professional help: Jordan, United Arab Emirates (UAE) and Arabs in Israel. *International Journal of Social Psychiatry*, 50(2), 102–114.

Brinson, J. A., & Al-Amri, F. S. S. (2005). Students' perceptions of mental health counseling in the United Arab Emirates (UAE). *International Journal for the Advancement of Counselling*, 27(4), 495–512.

Dwairy, M. A. (2006). *Counseling and psychotherapy with Arabs and Muslims: A culturally sensitive approach*. New York: Teachers College Press.

Gladding, S. T. (2014). *Family therapy: History, theory, and practice*. Boston, MA: Pearson Higher Ed.

Klyukanov, I. (2005). *Principles of intercultural communication*. Boston, MA: Pearson College Division.

Koenig, H. G., Al Zaben, F., Sehlo, M. G., Khalifa, D. A., Al Ahwal, M. S., Qureshi, N. A., & Al-Habeeb, A. A. (2014). Mental health care in Saudi Arabia: Past, present and future. *Open Journal of Psychiatry*, 4(2), 113.

Qureshi, N. A., Al-Habeeb, A. A., & Koenig, H. G. (2013). Mental health system in Saudi Arabia: An overview . *Neuropsychiatr Dis Treat*, 9(1121), 35.

Rasheed, A. A. (2015). The lived experiences of international counselor education students during their field-based clinical supervision in the United States of America. (Doctoral dissertation). Duquesne University.

Sewilam, A. M., Watson, A. M., Kassem, A. M., Clifton, S., McDonald, M. C., Lipski, R., … & Nimgaonkar, V. L. (2015). Suggested avenues to reduce the stigma of mental illness in the Middle East. *International Journal of Social Psychiatry*, 61(2), 111–120.

Triandis, H. C. (1993). Collectivism and individualism as cultural syndromes. *Cross-cultural Research*, 27(3–4),155–180.

World Health Organization. Department of Mental Health, & Substance Abuse. (2014). *Mental health atlas 2014*. London: World Health Organization.

13

FAMILIAS FUERTES

Strength-Based Approaches to Working with Latino Immigrant Families

E. Carolina Benitez and Daniel Gutierrez

Introduction

Over 55 million individuals of Latino origin reside in the United States, accounting for 17% of the total population (U.S. Census Bureau, 2014a). Thirty-six percent of Latinos living in the United States are foreign-born (U.S. Census Bureau, 2014a). As the fastest growing racial/ethnic minority group in the United States, Latinos are projected to make up about 31% of the total US population by 2050 (U.S. Census Bureau, 2014b). In fact, several states expect their Latino population to continue to steadily increase and even dominate the current portrait of their population much sooner: Texas by 2027 and California by 2042.

Latinos face a number of challenges as they transition from their country of origin, including an increased pressure to acculturate and assimilate, exposure to hardships and poverty related to immigrating, and experiencing negative reception from the host culture. Although for Latinos the decision to immigrate to the United States is less often associated with a desire to pursue luxuries, and more often associated with a duty to meet the most essential needs of the family, the process yields a number of life experiences and stressors that when left unaddressed and unresolved can lead to mental health complications. However, despite the need for services, the Surgeon's General report on mental health estimates that fewer than 1 in 11 Latinos suffering from mental health disorders receive specialized services and fewer than 1 in 5 receive these services even within a primary care setting (Department of Health and Human Services [DHHS], 2001).

The lack of culturally and linguistically suitable mental health services keeps many Latinos suffering with mental illness from seeking services. Additionally, there is a limited number of providers who can offer bilingual or bicultural services, resulting in miscommunication and, perhaps more importantly, misunderstandings in assessment, diagnosis, and treatment planning. However, language barriers affect more than what takes place in the counseling office; Latinos who are not proficient in English also have limited access to critical information about how and where to access services, as well as with completing the mandatory (and extensive) paperwork required at clinics.

There are a number of additional systemic factors that influence the underutilization of mental health services for Latinx families. For example, stigma plays a critical role, and so does documentation status, a fear of deportation for foreign-born Latinx, and a mistrust of the system. To explore each one of these factors would go beyond the scope of this chapter and add too many pages to read. Therefore, we will turn our attention now to Latino family culture.

Cultural Factors Affecting Mental Health

Latino Family Structure

Family life in the United States has continued to undergo significant changes, including an increase in age at marriage, cohabitation trends, the number of children born outside of marriage, and an increase in more female-led families. Latinos living in the USA have also seen important changes in their family structure. This is an important factor to consider related to how Latino individuals and families access resources, including mental health services. Since family life and relationships is central to Latino culture, it is vital to understand the nature of family life among Latinos. As mentioned before, clinicians must consider how the immigration experience may have affected Latino family structure through acculturation and intermarriage. This new shaping within an ethnic population often leads to a blurring of ethnic/cultural boundaries.

Gender Roles

The cultural norms and expectations that Latinos are exposed to have singular effects on their mental health. For example, Latino women report higher rates of depressive and anxiety disorders than do Latino men. Some believe that perhaps the added pressures of balancing traditional role expectations of their native culture and new roles delineated by the US culture may act as a risk factor for psychiatric disorders. However, in regard to substance use, Latino women are at an advantage when compared to Latino men and their US born counterparts, due in part to traditional views that frown upon female substance use. Additionally, Latino women enjoy a strong cultural identity and obligation rooted in family values that may provide for some women a sense of purpose and meaning. When working with Latino men, clinicians should seek to explore social roles, supports, and stressors and how these may be linked to their risk of mental illness. Traditional gender roles among Latino men place them at the center of financial obligations within the family, which can also function as a protective factor when it provides meaning, and as a risk factor when it causes distress instead. For example, a husband who suddenly finds himself out of the workforce may become at risk for depressive disorders, while his ability to provide for the family may contribute to better mental health outcomes.

Machismo and Marianismo

Gender socialization is very complex in the Latino culture, influenced in great part by the immigration and acculturation process. Early literature suggests that gender relations were mainly patriarchal, especially in rural settings were a clear division of labor demarcated male and female activities inside and outside the home. Historically, Latino men have been charged with financially supporting the family and Latina women with caring for the home and children. However, urbanization, migration, and industrialization transformed patriarchal arrangements. Latinas, especially those living in the United Stated, have expanded their spatial mobility and joined the workforce, albeit not necessarily decreasing the domestic responsibilities typically assigned to females. Therefore, although marianismo and machismo are values that inform behavior, the patterns of behavior themselves can and do still vary.

Marianismo is a concept that is based on the Catholic ideal of the Virgin Mary and that emphasizes women's role as mothers. Within this role, self-sacrifice and suffering for the children and family well-being are respected and celebrated. Due to this primary obligation to the family, women were often restricted. However, in the USA, Latina women have moved towards more egalitarian gender roles within the family and society after securing work outside the home. Often times, traditional values within the Latino culture, including the importance of religion and church attendance, are still passed down by the female figure. However, the ideology of patriarchy and machismo has been challenged and Latina females have stepped into traditionally male-dominated positions, like farm working and construction, but also achieving greater success academically and professionally.

In contrast, machismo stresses the male role of a head of household, not of a father. Depending on the perspective and context, machismo has been viewed under both a positive and negative lens. Feminists who have challenged the traditional roles of gender within Latino culture have identified machismo as amplified masculinity and male chauvinism. For others, machismo describes a role that historically helped Latino families preserve family pride and respect.

Although generally viewed as a stereotype, Latino machismo and gender relations overall have been documented (Alvirez & Bean, 1976; Mummert, 1993). However, feminist reinterpretations in the last decades have greatly contributed to our understanding of Latino families and offered a broader lens under which to explore gender roles. For example, they have examined and reinterpreted the functions of machismo and offered a glance into its positive aspects, including appreciating men as protectors and providers.

Family Education and Employment

In the United States, Latino children typically live with a parent or guardian who is less educated than their white counterpart. According to Pew Research Center, in the 2016 elections an estimated 83% (2016) of Latino families cited education as very important to their vote. However, finances continue to be the main obstacle for Latinos to enroll in college. The same source cited a 2014 National Journal poll which noted that 66% of Latinos interviewed who either enrolled in the military or joined the workforce directly after high school did so because supporting their family preceded other obligations; this compared to 39% of whites. Ethnic disparities in the US education system have long been a challenge for minorities.

In addition to finances, documentation status is a main determinant for education completion as well. An undocumented status precludes immigrants from accessing various public services, including those related to employment, health, and education. A very common and disturbing theme heard among Latino undocumented youth begins to reverberate around the time they gain awareness of their "illegality." For many, this happens when high school students approach graduation and are unable to follow in their peers' footsteps in the college selection process. While many Latino students excel academically and in extracurricular activities, without the proper documentation, higher education can be firmly out of reach. Without legal status, not only are Latino youth unable to apply to most colleges, the few which accept undocumented students are likely to charge out-of-state tuition regardless of state residence.

Cultural Strengths

Cultural Values

Cultural differences among individuals must be recognized in order to create an effective match between those who deliver services and their clients. There are three important cultural values that have been emphasized in research in terms of their potential to influence mental health outcomes for Latinos: *familismo, personalismo*, and *respeto*. Ideally, each of these values is implemented into models of prevention and early intervention for Latinos.

Familismo

For Latinos, the contributions of the extended family are an essential part of individual and family wellness (Cabassa, 2007; Snowden, 2007). As such, this cultural value focuses on family cohesion and is a critical factor for providers to consider when working with Latino clients and families. In order to assess mental health help-seeking behaviors among Latinos, researchers and providers alike are called to also evaluate the extent to which the role of family support impacts the individual's perception of their presenting problem. For example, Latino clients may approach the counseling office only after being told by family members/ friends to seek professional help. In other words, self-perception *and* family/social perception of need for care are both important predictors of service use, and, perhaps, of engagement. Consequently, Latinos in need of services may be more receptive to the advice of friends, family, and community leaders whom they trust and confide in.

Personalismo

A way of being and interacting within interpersonal relationships, personalismo is central to Latino culture. This personal approach to communications emphasizes warmth and leads to trust. Therapists who recognize the importance of honoring the cultural value of personalismo may find themselves venturing outside of expected ethical behavior for providers. For example, Latino clients often times expect some level of self-disclosure from their therapist before themselves opening up. Likewise, acceptance of small gifts and physical touch are also elements of personalismo that are important to developing and maintaining a therapeutic alliance that is built on trust. Practitioners offering culturally sensitive therapy should be prepared to have their conceptions about what constitutes elements of dual-relationships challenged. By accepting either, and always within the proper ethical boundaries, therapists are contributing to the preservation and strengthening of the alliance and exhibiting multicultural competency.

Respeto

The value of respeto customarily places emphasis on authority figures within and outside of the family. For example, ultimate decision-making power is given to parents, grandparents, and other elders, but also to teachers, healthcare providers, and government officials. In counseling, the client may be hesitant to disagree, express doubt or concern, or even speak up about their confusion related to any or all parts of the treatment process. In some cases, even attrition may be likelier than bringing questions to the therapist. The mutual regard that develops between Latino consumers and their providers requires that therapists gain an understanding of the hierarchical system within the culture. Therefore, providers will benefit from paying particular attention, during the assessment and throughout treatment, to the established structure as it relates to gender or generational hierarchy. Therapists who wish to work with Latinos and ensure compliance with treatment and retention must use active listening skills as well as ask questions to ensure that he or she has a clear picture of the client's individual perspective and experience regarding this and other important values.

In the context of families, respeto emphasizes obedience and delineates the boundaries between children and parents. Cross-cultural studies (Harwood, 1992; Harwood, Schoelmerich, Schulze, & Gonzalez, 1999) have observed, for example, that Latino parents are more likely to socialize their children to be respectful by asserting parental authority, discourage autonomy and exploration, and use physical restraint. By comparison, their white counterparts model, praise, and suggest as opposed to using direct mediations in parenting. Clinicians will need to adjust their own views of parenting and be able to incorporate more traditional Latino views into interventions.

Religion and Spirituality

It has long been established that religion and spirituality can provide support and help individuals and families deal with different challenges, including mental health conditions. According to the Pew Research Center (2017), about 55% of Latino adults identify as Catholic, 22% as Protestant, and less than 18% are religiously unaffiliated or identify with other non-Christian religions. Although these numbers continue to change as Latinos continue the journey of acculturation, 91% of Latinos state that religion is important to them.

In addition to ascribing to mainstream religions, many Latino subgroups also include elements of spiritual and folk healing. *Curanderos, Santeros*, and *Espiritistas* represent folk healers and religious/spiritual belief systems. *Curanderos* are often called on to treat physical, mental, or spiritual ailments using herbal remedies, messages, and cleansing rituals. *Santeros* are also folk healers, and blend African and Catholic beliefs usually practiced by Cubans and other Caribbean ethnic groups. *Espiritistas* are healers who primarily treat mental illness and is a term used primarily by Puerto Ricans. This belief system includes reincarnation and mediums. Latinos are likely to seek help from primary care providers for most illnesses, including mental and emotional concerns, but in many cases, they may also turn to clergy and folk/spiritual healers in conjunction with or as an alternative to Western care. Therefore, clinicians must be informed about how Latino cultural values and attitudes are often heavily influenced by spiritual beliefs.

Strength-Based Family Counseling

Standard models of counseling practiced in the United States tend to emphasize deficits and disorders, and often value traits that can feel incongruent with the worldview of Latinos (Parra-Cardona, Córdova, Holtrop, Escobar-Chew, & Horsford, 2009). As previously mentioned in this book, too often, culture is used as a method of cataloging clients into broad categories, and this process tends to lead to gross generalizations and (unintentional) further marginalization. Thus, clinicians should not ignore the unique and multi-layered dimensions of the Latino ethnic identity. Instead, therapists must adopt approaches to counseling that are culturally responsive and emphasize Latino values and strengths. Strength-based approaches help reduce stigma and empower families to use existing resources to achieve their goals. Additionally, counseling interventions that are adapted to align with a client's cultural values are four times more effective than typical approaches (Griner & Smith, 2006). In the following section, we briefly outline some of the strength-based approaches we recommend for working with Latino families.

Deconstructing Latino Family Dimensions

The first step in working with Latino families is most likely going to be conducting a thorough assessment. From a strength-based perspective, the assessment process is about getting to know, understand, and join with the family. When working with Latino families it is important to begin by deconstructing the dimensions of identity. Pioneering counselor in Latino mental health, Patricia Arredondo, developed the Latino Dimensional of Personal Identity (DPI) model to help counselors and helping professionals better understand and explore Latino family identity (Arredondo & Santiago-Rivera, 2000). Arredondo's model categorizes aspects of Latino identity into three dimensions (A, B, & C): (1) the A dimension represents factors of identity that are unchangeable, like demographic characteristics, such as age, gender, language; (2) the B dimension represents factors that are a little more under the individual's control but are directly influenced by A and C, and are less visible, such as acculturation level, educational level, geographic location, economic status, recreational interests; and (3) the C dimension includes socio-political events that influence the family in such a way that they are embedded in their identity, such as the history of colonialization, immigration policies, war, etc. For more information on the ABC dimensional model we recommend the seminal work by Arredondo & Santiago-Rivera (2000). The goal of the model is to ensure that counselors do not overlook important aspects of Latino identity. Oftentimes, the intake process with a family barely explores any deeper than the demographic information. However, only assessing demographic information fails to bring to light factors that could be critical to family counseling. For example, the life experiences and stress level of a Latino family who recently immigrated to the USA as an attempt to escape war is going to be considerably different than a Latino born in Puerto Rico (a US territory).

Marriage and Relationship Education

Marriage and relationship education is a psycho-educational approach designed to strengthen family relationships and foster healthy family functioning (Hawkins et al., 2008). There are many evidence-based MRE programs and each has their own unique angle and approach, but the majority of these programs use curricula designed to serve as preventive interventions by teaching skills and strategies that mitigate problems before they get worse (Hawkins et al., 2008). Gutierrez et al. (2014) noted several significant benefits associated with using MRE with Latino families in the USA. First, MRE interventions are cost-effective. Due to the lack of healthcare insurance in the Latino community, cost of service is a significant barrier to care. MRE is typically offered in group formats and serves as a preventive intervention which allows for costs to be kept low. MRE is also culturally flexible. Many MRE curriculums are available in Spanish (see www.prepinc.com), and there is research to support their use with Latino families. Because MRE is skills-based and done in a group setting it aligns with the Latino cultural values of personalismo and helps alleviate some of the stigma around seeking traditional family counseling services. Lastly, many (if not most) MRE programs are designed to be facilitated by lay helpers in church settings. There are several faith-based MRE programs, and these programs tend to draw the interest of the many Latino families that are strongly rooted in their faith tradition.

Brief Family Counseling Approaches

The duration of a counseling session and the length of treatment will always depend upon the family and the presenting concern, and many Latino families may prefer long-term therapy approaches, such as in Argentina where psychoanalysis is preferred and in high demand. However, there are many reasons why Latino families in the USA and their counselors would prefer to utilize a brief family counseling approach. For instance, brief counseling may seem more inviting to someone who is still coping with feelings related to stigma, or for someone who is struggling with economic hardships and is tentative about committing to long-term treatment. Brief counseling is also more likely to be consistent with Latino perceptions of health care (e.g., more akin to medical care with a family physician).

Two of the oldest family therapy approaches that can be adapted for brief therapy include Jay Hayley's Strategic Family Counseling and Salvador Minuchin's Structural Family Therapy. These approaches focus on the relationships between family members, and the various dynamics within the family system, emphasizing treatment on re-balancing power throughout a family, establishing healthy boundaries, and fostering family communication and cohesion through directive intervention. There is limited research on adapting these approaches for Latino families but their emphasis on hierarchy, power, and systems is consistent with Latino cultural values (Szapocznik & Kurtines, 1993; Zafra, 2016).

Another strength-based approach recommended for Latino families is the Integrated Model for Brief Couples Counseling (IMBCC; Gutierrez, Carlson, Daire, & Young, 2017; Long & Young, 2006; Young & Carlson, 2011). The IMBCC is a five stage brief couples counseling model that allows for therapist to be eclectic in their approach but keep the format of brief counseling. In short, the IMBCC involves doing a thorough clinical assessment of the family or couple, developing an interactive joint definition of the problem by using a technique known as *the big reframe* (O'Brien & Young, 2014), establishing goals for the couple or family, and selecting interventions that directly address each goal. When the clients have met their goal, counseling moves on to developing strategies for maintaining change and validating the outcomes. Gutierrez et al. (2017) found the IMBCC to be effective in increasing relationship satisfaction and reducing mental health symptomology in a sample of low-income and distressed couples. The IMBCC can be especially beneficial for families who have limited resources and are struggling with significant issues as is the case for many Latino immigrants.

The Immigrant Narrative Using Genograms

The immigrant journey is a critical part of the Latino immigrant experience. Oftentimes, novice counselors are worried about discussing topics related to immigration status for fear that it might become too politically charged or offensive. However, for most immigrants, migrating to the United States is a critical moment in their lives, and to not explore issues of immigration because of fear and trepidation would be to avoid truly connecting with a client's experience and daily reality. It is an error in practice to avoid a part of a family's experience because of your own feelings towards the topic. Thus, finding strategies for exploring and unpacking the family's immigration narrative is important.

One method of exploring generational issues in an immigrant family is to use a genogram. The genogram has a long history in marriage and family therapy, and is a central component of intergenerational and systemic approaches like Bowenian family therapy. The genogram allows for a symbolic representation of family hierarchy and relationships using an established set of shapes and figures. If you are a marriage and family therapist or one in training, it is likely you already know how to develop a genogram for a family. For further details on how to develop a genogram we recommend the seminal study by McGoldrick et al. (1999). When working with Latino families, one can adapt the genogram to include information about generational status (e.g., first generation, second, 1.5 generation, etc.), immigration status, language fluency, and connection with country of origin (e.g., close with extended family, distant, estranged). Family therapist could then use the genogram to explore family history and specifically address topics related to immigration and acculturation. Consider a family where parents are concerned about preserving family history while the child wishes to explore and "fit into" the new culture. By creating a genogram, family therapists can facilitate this discussion with the family and hopefully establish a mutual understanding among family members.

Case Example

Marcela and Felipe have been married for 14 years. They immigrated to Houston Texas from Nicaragua about 13 years ago. Felipe came to the United States on a work visa. Since living in the United States, they have had two children, Samuel, age 10 and Javier, age 12. Recently, Felipe has been struggling with a lot of anxiety and depression. He reports that he is anxious about some of the discriminatory comments he has been hearing at work, and the increase in anti-Latino rhetoric found in the news. Marcela has also felt a sense of anxiety about the news, and is concerned about her family, including her extended family in Nicaragua whom she has not seen since moving to the Texas. Marcela and Felipe also find themselves in constant conflict over parenting issues. Felipe worries that their children are "giving up their Latino roots" while Marcela thinks it is critical that they learn to blend in. Felipe also expresses concerns that he has done a horrible thing by taking his wife away from her family in Nicaragua, and that they will experience financial ruin.

Frustrated by the constant fighting and concerned about Felipe's health, Marcela asks her pastor for advice. Her pastor recommends that Felipe and Marcela take part in a Marriage and Relationship Education (MRE) program being hosted at the church. At first Marcela and Felipe are hesitant about attending, but they were encouraged because of their trust for their pastor and because they knew that the program would be brief and provide childcare. The MRE program teaches Marcela and Felipe useful skills related to communication and parenting. Felipe chooses not to talk much during the group, but he remarks after the first few sessions, that he found the information in the group very useful, and especially liked the informal and friendly nature of the instructor. At the end of the MRE groups, the couple was given the opportunity to take part in a few sessions of one-on-one family counseling. Marcela was excited about the opportunity, but Felipe was reluctant, and she would never push the issue with him. After meeting with the counselor at the MRE meetings, Felipe decided it would be worth a try. The counselor used the Integrated Model for Brief Couples Counseling as the framework for his work with Marcela and Felipe. He spent the first few sessions building the relationship and conducting a thorough assessment, using the immigrant genogram and deconstructing the Latino family dimensions. The family discussed their identity as Latinos and the counselor facilitated a discussion regarding acculturation, acculturative stress, and how identity is multifaceted and more than just country of origin. Using the communication skills learned in the MRE sessions, Felipe and Marcela began facilitating discussions with their kids and with each other. Felipe was relieved to hear that his children were still proud of their heritage even though they were trying to fit in with friends, and Marcela and Felipe were better able to manage their conflict. The family counselor encouraged the family to spend quality time together, suggesting a family game night, and setting apart time to eat dinner together each evening. Also, Felipe and Marcela were encouraged to share with their children the strengths of their culture and stories of life back in Nicaragua. After about six sessions, Felipe reported feeling closer to his family, especially Marcela. Marcela also reported that, although she still missed her family, it helped to know that she could talk to Felipe about her stress and share her stories of her family with her children.

Conclusions and Recommendations

The goal of this chapter is to present you with a description of Latino families living in the United States and offer practical strategies for working with these families. Of course, there is no one perfect approach that would work with all Latino families, but taking into account the various factors that influence Latino family functioning and mental health, and developing an understanding of Latino cultural values allows marriage and family counselors to adapt approaches to best serve Latino clients. Additionally, we shared several approaches (MRE, Brief Approaches) that are validated by experience and research to work well with Latinos. Finally, we provided a brief case study that demonstrated how to sequence these different techniques in a session with a Latino family.

References

Alvirez, D., & Bean, F. D. (1976). The Mexican American family. In C. H. Mindel & R. N. Haberstein (Eds.), *Ethnic families in America* (pp. 271–292). New York: Elsevier.

Arredondo, P., & Santiago-Rivera, A. (2000). Latino dimensions of personal identity (adapted from Personal Dimensions of Identity Model). Unpublished manuscript.

Cabassa, L. J. (2007). Latino immigrant men's perceptions of depression and attitudes toward help-seeking. *Hispanic Journal of Behavioral Sciences*, 29, 492–509.

Department of Health and Human Services. (2001). *Mental health: Culture, race, and ethnicity— A supplement to mental health: A report of the Surgeon General.* Rockville, MD: Substance Abuse and Mental Health Services Administration.

Griner, D. & Smith, T. B. (2006). Culturally adapted mental health interventions: A meta-analytic review. *Psychotherapy: Theory, Research, Practice, Training*, 43, 531–548.

Gutierrez, D., Barden, S. M., & Tobey, M. (2014). Mejorando matrimonios: Relationship education as a vehicle to overcome barriers for Hispanic couples. *The Family Journal*, 22, 148–155.

Gutierrez, D., Carlson, R. G., Daire, A. P., & Young, M. E. (2017). Evaluating treatment outcomes using the Integrative Model of Brief Couples Counseling: A pilot study. *The Family Journal*, 25, 1.

Harwood, R. L. (1992). The influence of culturally derived values on Anglo and Puerto Rican mothers' perceptions of attachment behavior. *Child Development*, 63(4), 822–839.

Harwood, R. L., Schoelmerich, A., Schulze, P. A., & Gonzalez, Z. (1999). Cultural differences in maternal beliefs and behaviors: A study of middle-class Anglo and Puerto Rican mother-infant pairs in four everyday situations. *Child Development*, 70(4), 1005–1016.

Hawkins, A. J., Blanchard, V. L., Baldwin, S. A., & Fawcett, E. B. (2008). Does marriage and relationship education work? A meta-analytic study. *Journal of Consulting & Clinical Psychology*, 76, 723–734.

Krogstad, J. M. (2016). Five facts about Latinos and education. Retrieved from www.pewresearch.org/fact-tank/2016/07/28/5-facts-about-latinos-and-education/.

Krogstad, J. M., & Passel, J. S. (2015). Five facts about illegal immigration in the U.S. Retrieved from www.pewresearch.org/fact-tank/2015/11/19/5-facts-about-illegal-immigration-in-the-u-s/.

Krogstad, J. M., Passel, J. S., & Cohn, D. (2017). Five facts about illegal immigration in the U.S. Retrieved from www.pewresearch.org/fact-tank/2017/04/27/5-facts-about-illegal-immigration-in-the-u-s/.

Long, L. L., & Young, M. E. (2006). *Counseling and therapy for couples* (2nd ed.). Belmont, CA: Thomson Brooks/Cole.

McGoldrick, M., Gerson, R., & Shellenberger, S. (1999). *Genograms: Assessment and intervention* (2nd ed.). New York: W. W. Norton & Company.

Mummert, G. (1993). Changes in the formation of western rural families: Profound modifications [Cambios en la formacióm de las familias rurales del Occidente: Modificaciones profundas]. *Demographic Studies*, 6, 23–24.

O'Brien, E. R., & Young, M. E. (2014). The big reframe: Helping couples develop an interactive definition. *The Family Journal*, 22(3), 347–349. http://dx.doi.org/10.1177/1066480714533655.

Parra-Cardona, J., Córdova, D., & Holtrop, K. (2009). Culturally informed emotionally focused therapy with latino/a immigrant couples. In M.Rastogi & V. Thomas (Eds.), *Multicultural couple therapy* (pp. 345–368). Thousand Oaks, CA: SAGE.

Snowden, L. R. (2007). Explaining mental health treatment disparities: Ethnic and cultural differences in family involvement. *Culture, Medicine, and Psychiatry*, 31(3), 389–402.

Smart, J. F., & Smart, D. W. (1995). Acculturative stress of Hispanics: Loss and challenge. *Journal of Counseling & Development*, 73(4), 390–396. Retrieved from http://search.proquest.com/docview/219029338?accountid=14605.

Szapocznik, J., & Kurtines, W. M. (1993). Family psychology and cultural diversity: Opportunities for theory, research, and application. *American Psychologist*, 48(4), 400–407.

U.S. Census Bureau. (2014a). American fact finder: Hispanic or Latino origin [Data file]. Retrieved from http://factfinder.census.gov/faces/.

U.S. Census Bureau. (2014b). American fact finder: Hispanic or Latino origin [Data file]. Retrieved from www.census.gov/data/tables/2014/demo/popproj/2014-summary-tables.html.

U.S. Census Bureau. (2015). American fact finder: Hispanic or Latino origin [Data file]. Retrieved from www.census.gov/newsroom/facts-for-features/2015/cb15-ff18.html.

Young, M. E., & Carlson, R. G. (2011). Fragile families, fragile couples. *Counseling and Human Development*, 43(7), 1–12.

Zafra J. (2016). The use of structural family therapy with a Latino family: A case study. *Journal of Systemic Therapies*, 35(4), 11–21.

14

CULTURALLY CONTEXTUAL FAMILY THERAPY WITH INVOLUNTARY CLIENTS

Bethany Simmons and Jamie Banker

Introduction

Involuntary clients, who represent a broad category of diverse populations, present unique challenges and contexts for clinicians. Increasingly, clients are referred, coerced, or mandated to participate in counseling by family members or other larger social systems, rather than requesting counseling voluntarily. This produces new implications for clinical work. Many of the challenges of conducting counseling and utilizing traditional psychotherapy approaches with involuntary clients have minimally been addressed in the family counseling and marriage and family therapy literature (Haley, 1997; Lipchik, 2002; Snyder & Anderson, 2009; Sotero, Cuhna, Silva, Escudero, & Relvas, 2016). It is necessary to consider the systemic, cultural, relational, and contextual elements that can enhance counseling work with these clients.

Effectively engaging involuntary clients in counseling requires clinicians to be mindful of the intricate complexity related to cultural contexts. This is especially true because involuntary clients are often ethnically diverse, underserved, marginalized, under-resourced, and in positions of less power and privilege. Clinicians also need to be aware of the interaction between multiple cultural systems and social justice issues that influence both the client's and the counselor's lives (Baker, 1999; Friedlander, Escudero, & Heatherington, 2006; Lipchik, 2002). These cultural diversity and social justice issues can be connected to clients' attendance and participation in counseling, presenting complaints, goals, and possible solutions.

Systemic focused treatments lead to a contextually tailored approach that invites culturally diverse involuntary clients to engage in the counseling process. The authors have found this to be true across diverse settings and various types of involuntary clients (e.g. judicial, legal, medical, social services, psychiatric facilities, family counseling, couples counseling, child/adolescent counseling). Systemically oriented counselors understand the significance and influence of relationships, not only in the client's immediate family life but also those they are a part of in larger societal systems. And, family counselors understand they too are in relationship with the client, and it is that relationship which provides the foundation and fertile ground for any counseling work.

Family counselors have to be aware of not only their relationships with their clients but also their role in their client's larger social system. This becomes complex when clients are not necessarily seeking counseling on their own fruition and may even be coerced. The authors invite family counselors to learn how to identify an involuntary client, to think about the complexity of working with involuntary clients, provide areas of focus for treatment, and offer culturally sensitive strategies and systemic tools for a family-based cultural contextual approach for working with involuntary clients.

Who Is an Involuntary Client?

While involuntary clients represent a broad category, they all have in common that they are not seeking treatment voluntarily. The most common definition of involuntary clients are clients seeking treatment because someone else requires them to attend or else they will face significant and well-defined consequences. Another category, that can easily be overlooked, is nonvoluntary clients who are pressured or directed to attend treatment in more covert ways. Therefore, involuntary clients are often distinguished into two categories: those who are legally mandated by a social system such as by the court, child protective services, or other community agencies; and those nonvoluntary clients pressured to attend by others such as a spouse, parent, school, or employer (Rooney, 2009; Sotero, Major, Escudero & Relvas, 2016). Those who appear to be volunteering to attend counseling, but are only doing so because they are being told they must attend in order to prevent or avoid negative ramifications, we describe as "voluntold" clients. Involuntary clients seeking counseling is prevalent and it is likely that a portion of a family counselor's work will be with involuntary clients. We find that involuntary clients fall into one of these seven categories outlined in Table 14.1.

Who Mandates Counseling?

We refer to those who are requiring or strongly suggesting counseling of another person as the mandator throughout this chapter (even if they are not legally mandating treatment). A mandator of counseling is someone with an invested interest in the outcome of the counseling (not just the individual(s) seeking counseling), who requires/pressures attendance and seeks change in the person(s)

TABLE 14.1 Seven Categories of Involuntary Clients

Category of Involuntary Client	*Mandator*	*Examples*
1. *Those under someone else's care/holds healthcare decision-making power*	Counseling services may be prompted by caretaker or others involved who may have to consent for treatment	Most children, adolescents, elderly, disabled, medical, or severe mental illness, foster care
2. *Someone not abiding by the law*	Courts, probation officer, legal system	DWI/DUI, drug use/distribution, child/elder/disabled adult abuse/neglect, assault, domestic violence, sex crimes, stealing, etc.
3. *Someone in crisis or presenting bizarre, disruptive, or potentially harmful behavior*	Courts, legal system, mental health professionals, families	Exhibiting psychotic symptoms, suicidal/homicidal intent or attempt, threatening/aggressive actions are often mandated to therapy for the protection of self or others
4. *Someone not fulfilling/following the expectations/rules of a social system*	Schools, employers, military, medical, or psychiatric hospitals, government entities	Many of these cases involve "voluntold" clients, such as those experiencing: difficulty with an employer or work environment, inability to focus/obey in school classroom, difficulty completing expected tasks of system, difficulty continuing military duties, etc.
5. *Someone not fulfilling/following the expectations/rules of an interpersonal system*	Partner/spouse/family member mandating treatment or face the termination or change of the relationship	Anyone in relationships
6. *Someone wanting/needing to receive benefits or medical attention/care/services*	Insurance companies, medical professionals, government entities, legal system	Surgical procedures, managed care to pay for auxiliary services/medication and eligibility to receive disability or social security benefits may require counseling for the client receive benefits or medical attention, care, and services
7. *Ambiguous mandate*	Anyone	Clients are told they need to or are pressured to attend treatment and may be consequences if they do not obey this directive, but sometimes those consequences are unclear or undefined. This can lead to clients who are not only undecided about seeking treatment but also ambiguous about outcome

mandated to attend. The mandator is often in a position of power related to the client and in some instances the mandator requiring counseling may be an attempt to remediate or control the involuntary client's behavior or thinking. Because the client is at risk to lose something (e.g. freedom, their child, health, etc.) in this interdependent relationship, they may seek services to appease the mandator and prevent loss or avoid negative consequences. Conversely, there is benefit or gain for the mandating person/system(s) for the "client" to change through counseling. Many times, the motivation for the "client" to change rests with the mandator rather than the "client." The persuasion to attend counseling is often framed as in the "client's" best interest or to benefit the "client." Involuntary clients may not always see the benefit to treatment beyond avoiding more serious ramifications. Below we will highlight some of the unique challenges and characteristics of working with these clients.

Unique Challenges and Characteristics of Working with Involuntary Clients

Clients seeking treatment voluntarily differ drastically from those who do not. Yet, many counselors use the same counseling approaches that are predicated on the notion that the client is voluntarily participating in the counseling process and is seeking assistance as a way to create change in his or her life. Some of the unique challenges and characteristics of working with involuntary clients that family counselors may face in contrast to working with voluntary clients are outlined in Table 14.2.

TABLE 14.2 Unique Challenges and Characteristics of Involuntary Clients

Unique Challenges and Characteristics of Working with Involuntary Clients
Client is not there on their own initiative
Client may not desire or see a need for change. Someone else wants them to change
Client may be "punished" if he/she doesn't participate in treatment or meet expected outcomes of requiring system
Client may not want to be in treatment
Those mandating treatment have a stake in the outcome
Your "client" is more than just the person sitting in the therapy room – the term client also includes all those who want change and are requesting your help
Mandating person/system may want/require sharing of confidential information about treatment
Client may view you as an extension of the mandating system
Counselor may be "caught in the middle" and face dual relationships – with an obligation to involuntary client as well as to mandating persons/system
Building a relationship of trust with both the involuntary client and mandating persons/system
The counselor's role in the system involving the mandated client/mandating system – counselor may be an agent of social control

Intervention

As Haley (1997) pointed out, clinical work with involuntary clients requires a different, more systemic approach. A family-based cultural contextual approach to working with involuntary clients is informed by systemic family therapy clinical approaches (Becvar & Becvar, 2013) and is attuned to each client's unique cultural/social/political/familial context, with consideration of social justice issues. We find that how the family counselor conceptualizes treatment with each client is not only assessment and treatment planning but also intervention. In the following section, we outline considerations for conceptualizing clinical work with this population, as well as strategies for intervening to promote engagement in counseling and the change process.

Developing a Cultural Contextual Framework

Dominant Culture Norms

The values, rules, and every structure of our societal system are organized to protect, accommodate, and benefit the dominant groups in society (McGoldrick & Hardy, 2008). It is important to recognize that "racial, sexist, cultural, classist, and heterosexist power hierarchies constrain our clients' lives and determine what gets defined as a problem and what services our society will set up to respond to these problems" (McGoldrick & Hardy, 2008, pp. 4–5). Family counselors should be aware of these power hierarchies that may be coercing clients into therapy or defining the problem and ultimately the goal or outcomes for them. For example, a first-generation working class Latino adolescent may be referred to therapy by his school because of his poor performance in school and his unengaged parents. However, the expectations at school may be based on white suburban middle-class norms. These norms do not apply to an adolescent who needs to help the family survive financially by working to make money during homework time or when the school is offering tutoring and extracurricular activities and the adolescent's parents cannot leave work to attend the parent-school meetings.

Issues of Social Justice

Just as with voluntary clients, counselors who are attuned to cultural factors have to also assess how these cultural factors relate to social justice issues. Sometimes the changes requested or required of the client may not be possible for the client to achieve or, in some circumstances the requests ignore the reality of the person's situation. For example, an African-American single mother of 10 children, employed by a minimum wage job and participating in a court-ordered program is sent to jail for 30 days for failure to pay probation fees totaling $100. The case manager, under direction of the court, now instructs the mother's counselor that financial management must be a part of her treatment plan as a requirement of completing her probation and court-order program. This mandate failed to consider the reality of this family's lack of resources, court fees she was also paying for one of her teenage sons in another court-ordered program for selling drugs that may have been supporting the family.

Family counselors should consider the following questions surrounding social justice issues when working with any involuntary case. Who is most invested in seeing change happen? In many cases, family counselors are not just answering to the person in the therapy room in front of them, but sometimes even more so to the others requiring the person's attendance. Does the "client" have an interest or investment in changing or in therapy? Is that change realistic or possible for them, even if they wanted to make changes? What are the possible benefits as well as risks for the client if they attend counseling or make changes? What are the benefits and risks for the mandating person/system(s) if the client does or does not change? Are there any unforeseen or unintended consequences that could arise for the client or mandator if change does/doesn't happen? Is the counselor being asked to be an agent of social control to shape socially desired behavior and thinking? Whom is the counselor actually working for? Are they working for the mandating person/system(s), the client, or both? The counselor should be aware of their own values, judgments, and biases surrounding working with involuntary clients and the issues they present. It is important for counselors to recognize who they are aligning with in these counseling systems whether they are aware of it or not.

Social Constraints and the Larger Social System

Involuntary clients, family counselors, and mandating person/system(s) often find themselves in "double-bind" situations (Bateson, Jackson, Weakland, & Haley, 1956), where they are caught between contradictory requests/demands, which are impossible to respond to with all parties, and will evoke serious consequences if they are not responded to. To go back to our earlier example of the single-mother family, in order to help his family have food and survive, her son sells drugs. He has to choose between protecting his family for survival and the legal system/society's need for the youth to follow laws to protect the larger public. Further, despite maximizing government assistance and working night-shift hours, in order to help her teenage son follow the law, the mother may take on additional work, which then creates the problem of providing childcare for her toddlers during the day. The mother's inability to provide both financially and parentally for her family, the son's at-risk illegal activity and the court's responses are all embedded within a larger social/political/cultural context. Furthermore, this family is also impacted by racial and social class disparities in the distribution of and access to resources and increased incarceration rates with harsher court penalization for African Americans (McGoldrick & Hardy, 2008).

In this case, if the mother and son respond to protect their family and provide for their survival, they fail the court system and ultimately may end up in jail. If they meet the demands of the court, they fail their family and risk losing them. If the legal system does not intervene, they put the public at risk and if the family counselor cannot assist the family to make changes, they put the family and the public at risk. It is critical that family counselors assess their client's entire system including the larger social system and recognize the social constraints placed on all participants within the larger system (including on the counselor). If family counselors do not attend to the larger social issues, they become focused on the individual. However, often a client's ability to change is connected to his or her larger social systems and outside of their control.

This can be particularly challenging for family counselors when ethical, legal, and therapeutic dilemmas conflict with each other. For instance, it is common for involuntary clients or their counselors to be required to share information about treatment with the mandating party. Despite counselors' legal and ethical obligation to protect confidentiality for counseling to be successful, it may be a requirement of the client's participation in counseling to sign consent that confidential information is shared (even if it is just attendance and progress in treatment). This conflict between what is required to fulfill the mandator's requirements doesn't line up with ethical codes (such as confidentiality) or what would be therapeutic for the person (creating a therapeutic context safe to divulge honestly), yet is expected for treatment to take place and for the client to avoid serious consequences if they do not consent. Family counselors must be very intentional about how they handle such expectations with all parties so that they are still maintaining ethical integrity surrounding their work with clients.

Treatment Planning Considerations

The family counselor should assess how cultural and social justice factors are ingrained within the context for treatment. When counseling involuntary individuals, couples, and families, at minimum, thinking and inquiry into the following areas should include where cultural and social justice considerations overlap with: 1) the reason and purpose for treatment; 2) the mandate/request for counseling; 3) the worldview/values/beliefs of both the "client" and mandating person/system(s); 4) both client and mandator, as well as the counselor's, assumptions, expectations, agendas, and desired outcome; 5) how does the system of counseling fit into the culture of the "client" or of the mandating person/system(s)?; 6) the "client's" motivation and willingness to engage in treatment/change; 7) how are larger social/political/relational cultural factors at play in this situation?; 8) how are family members' dynamics and family culture at play in this situation?; 9) what is the counselor's role in both micro and macro systems?

Strategies for Engagement and Intervention

Developing Relationships and Building Trust

With any client, developing the therapeutic relationship and connecting with clients is essential to engaging clients in the change process (Minuchin & Fishman, 1981) and effective outcomes (Hubble, Duncan, & Miller, 1999). While it is imperative, it is particularly challenging when it comes to working with involuntary clients (Corey, 2017; Sotero, Cuhna, Silva, Escudero, & Relvas, 2016). Research on the therapeutic relationship with involuntary clients stresses the significance of a) focusing on developing the relationship from the outset of treatment and continual monitoring throughout, b) prioritizing the client's perspective on the pressure and mandate to attend, c) creating structure and guidelines to promote safety and confidentiality for all participants to engage honestly, d) intervening to manage family interpersonal hostility and conflicts, e) helping family members have a sense of shared purpose, f) understanding what would make counseling worth it to attend and participate, g) not imposing goals or tasks without collaboration and commitment from participants, h) being aware of differing motivation, desires, and readiness for therapy among family members, i) "meeting clients where they are" and going slow, and j) taking account of cultural issues (Baker, 1999; Friedlander, Escudero, & Heatherington, 2006; Lipchik 2002, Snyder & Anderson, 2009; Sotero, Cuhna et al., 2016; Sotero, Major et al., 2016).

In addition, it is important to develop a therapeutic alliance with all parties and to avoid split-alliances (Lebow & Black, 2012). With involuntary clients, this requires developing multiple relationships at various levels simultaneously, between individuals and subsystems (Sotero, Cuhna et al., 2016; Sotero, Major et al., 2016; Snyder & Anderson, 2009). When working with individuals, this might mean exploring conjoint counseling sessions with family members or asking the probation officer to have a meeting with the counselor and client together. At the very least, the counselor should attempt to collaborate with other invested parties/systems by inviting all involved into the counseling process whether through consultation, collaboration, or into the treatment itself. Maintaining neutrality (Palazzoli, Boscolo, Cecchin, & Prata, 1978) or multipartiality (Anderson & Gehart, 2007) with all participants (both inside the counseling room and out) is essential when working systemically and collaboratively with multiple parties, especially with conjoint therapies and involuntary clients (Sotero, Major et al., 2016).

The family counselor should be very clear about their role and relationships with and to all parties, as well as explicitly discuss how they will be interacting with each party and the information they will or will not share. They should not appear to the client as another part of the mandating system/person(s) or as an authority figure. If the role of the counselor is truly to be a second arm of the court, for example, the counselor should be upfront about the expectation from the court of the counselor with their client, rather than appear they are only working on behalf of the client.

How the family counselor interacts with all parties raises some legal and ethical issues to be considered. For example, how does the family counselor collaborate with all parties and remain neutral, when ethical codes expect the counselor to be working for the client? Or, conversely, how does the counselor work for the client if they are contracted by an outside system? If the client is mandated by an outside system that requires sharing confidential information in order for the client to participate (e.g., and the client chooses to attend to avoid harsher consequences – and legally, they have given permission for the counselor to share information with the system), how can the family counselor still protect the client's right to confidentiality and participate with the mandating body as contracted or expected? The family counselor must be very clear with all parties and very intentional about what and how they share information. As Brodsky (2011) recommends, the counselor should be upfront and directive about the client's situation, rather than utilizing traditional counseling inquiry and asking a lot of questions, which could ironically feel more intrusive and pressuring to the client.

There are ways that counselors can work systemically with all parties in the best interest of all involved, even when there are competing views or interests. And, when it is clear to all involved that the counselor cannot change others, only each person can change themselves, it is implied that the counselor is there to support clients' efforts and responsibility for solutions, not be the agent of change for them (Lipchik, 2002).

A Cultural Contextual Focus and Working with All Systems

While true for all clients, within involuntary treatment, a culturally informed practitioner should approach each "client" as unique, with a unique context and culture that includes an understanding and acknowledgement of the influence of the complex cultural elements of their lived experience and the larger systems they are a part of. By being cognizant of the context clients are in, the counselor can begin to understand how client's behavior (and other person(s)/system(s) in the client's life) makes sense in that context, a cornerstone of systemic family therapy (Boszormenyi-Nagy & Framo, 1965). Focusing on each client's unique cultural contextual circumstances will promote the counselor's understanding of the client's perspective; any apprehension to engaging in counseling or change; pressure from outside forces that may be encouraging or preventing change; how to relate to the client and others involved; and what direction and framework to take in culturally sensitive and informed ways. A blanket approach to all involuntary clients is not only ill-informed, but does not respect each unique person(s) involved. Interventions should be contextual and mindful of cultural considerations. For example, if a counselor intervenes in such a way or suggests tasks that are counter to the client's culture or culture of the mandating party, failure is certain. Best case scenario in this situation, the client may avoid the task or be resistant, worst case scenario, the counselor could actually put the client at further risk if not accounting for contextual cultural elements of their particular circumstances.

One way family counselors can focus on clients' unique cultural context is to identify and understand the patterns of interaction, rules, coalitions, hierarchies, and cultural values of the multiple systems involved (Minuchin & Fishman, 1981). Counseling and interventions should align within those parameters and the counselor can then determine how to promote second-order changes (if possible) across systems (Watzlawick, Weakland, & Fisch, 1974). For example, the court perceives the client as "bad." How can the counselor help the client engage in behaviors that court would consider "good" to start creating new patterns of interaction with the court that the client would be open and receptive to trying that they would also see as beneficial? When designing tasks and interventions from a cultural contextual approach, the counselor should think about: how might they be perceived by the client (including family members)? Would they be intuitive or logical to the client's worldview/belief system/values? Is the client likely to do them? Is it realistic or practical for them? Could the intervention make things worse in their relationships with other systems/others? Or, could they even be potentially dangerous? (i.e., stop selling drugs – drug supplier that lives in their neighborhood comes after them and their family; stop working to focus on school – family is in danger of not having food to survive).

Throughout sessions, family counselors should be attuned to systemic dynamics. This includes recognizing the client's abilities and limitations within their context, such as social forces that are outside of their ability to change or control. It is useful to assume that 1) all people are doing the best they can within their given context and set of relationships, 2) client's behavior and responses reflect their assessment of how best to respond to their relationships and context, 3) client's behavior and responses make sense in their context (Ray, 2016) – all hallmarks of family systems practice. Are there ways the family counselor can help facilitate further strides/improvement in directions *both* the client and mandator desire? Or help the client work in collaboration *with* the mandator rather than in an oppositional relationship?

Expanding the definition of the problem beyond the individual to include the other person/system(s) involved allows all to begin to view the presenting concerns in a more complex and systemic manner (Micucci, 2009). It can also make clearer what is within each individual's control to alter and what is not. This can not only place responsibility for change where it belongs but it can also reinforce clients' personal agency to see where it is possible for them to act to make a desirable difference and freedom from the pressure to change what they cannot. Making this explicit to all person/system(s) can also allow others involved (including the mandator) to begin viewing the mandated individual differently.

Working systemically also requires that family counselors pay attention to their own biases. It is vital that the counselor does not inadvertently align with parts of the system or systems over others based on their own views, ignorance, or biases. Given counselors also work in a social/political/cultural context, they should be mindful of how they listen to clients, whose story they buy into more, the language they use, the suggestions they make, etc., to ensure they do not participate in further disenfranchisement of those they treat. Often, these may take the form of microaggressions (Boden, n.d.), which could fall outside of the family counselor's awareness if they are not intentionally thoughtful about how they relate to their clients. They could also repeat isomorphic patterns of interaction with the client (e.g., the counselor treats the client like their father does; the counselor holds strong views about the client's lifestyle, therefore aligning with the mandator or family members against the client or other members of the system) and perpetuate the problems if not astute. From our view, it is an ethical imperative that family counselors recognize their participation in the various systems and understand their influence in a second-order cybernetic way (Becvar, Canfield & Becvar, 1997).

Case Example

Shifting into a clinical example, we hope to further illuminate these areas of consideration and provide specific areas for inquiry and strategies for a family-based cultural contextual approach for working with involuntary clients. While this example is based on real clinical experience of the authors in various settings, the case is a combination of multiple clients and some constructed narrative and therefore do not include any identifying confidential information.

Vignette

During the first session with Vali, a 21-year-old woman attending a large university, she states that she is fed up with her mother who is controlling and over-intrusive in her life and the only reason she came to therapy was to avoid a fight with her mother. Vali says to you, "You know, you talked to her on the phone when she made the appointment for me." When Darci, Vali's mother, called, she stated that she was concerned about Vali's mood swings, mainly bouts of depression and anger, that culminate in Vali "being disrespectful to everyone in the home." After listening to Vali's mom, you invite them in for a family session. However, she did not oblige. She said, "there is nothing wrong with me or my family, Vali is the only one with a problem." At that time you informed Darci, that Vali must be the one to call and set up the appointment, which she did.

Vali says that her "mood swings," as her mother calls it, are just her way to express frustration with her parents about the rules and limits they put on her. She tells you that her parents are non-practicing Muslims from a conservative

Middle Eastern country, who moved to the US prior to having a family. Vali shares she has difficulty identifying with her family's culture since being born and raised in an urban US city. She describes herself as very Americanized. She indicates that, even though she was too young to remember, her parents share stories about some of the hate and discrimination they faced, particularly after September 11, 2001. She says that their fears have been raised with the recent US laws banning travel from her parents' country of origin.

During the session, Vali also tells you that she was raped when she was 17. She says that her parents were very ashamed of her and this situation because she had been drinking and they call her "damaged goods." Her parents made it clear that no one else but them should know about this, especially none of their family members, which made things complicated when Vali found out she was pregnant. She reports they convinced her to have an abortion and she still thinks about the abortion daily. She described the doctor's visits as "horrible" and felt they were judging her for her choices. Vali reports that her family doctor put her on some medications about six months after the incident due to some of the mood swings her mother reported to them. She says that starting college has helped her put her past behind her, but living at home is difficult and she looks forward to being able to move out sometime.

How to Proceed?

From a systemic perspective, we outline our suggested areas to consider, questions to explore, and ways to begin a family-based cultural contextual counseling approach with this "client." First and foremost, it is unclear whether Vali is a client interested in participating in counseling and returning for future sessions.

BOX 14.1 WORKING WITH VALI

Developing Relationships and Building Trust

Case Considerations

- How do Vali, Darci, other family members and society view my role as a counselor in this case?
- Do the laws of the state I practice in require me to report the rape if Vali reveals the person's name since she was a minor at the time, but is now an adult?
- If so, how could involving the legal system add more complexity to the work with Vali and the limits of confidentiality impair building a safe context and therapeutic relationship with Vali (and family) to participate in counseling, particularly in a social/political system where they have already experienced discrimination, and could reify cultural stigma and shame?

- On the other hand, how could not encouraging Vali to report the rape and treat "her problems" collude with gendered oppression, implying there is something wrong with her or that she shares equal responsibility for the incident rather than the perpetrator of violence (Tavris, 1992)?
- How can I treat Vali with honor, dignity, and respect to demonstrate it is her choice to participate in counseling or not and convey counseling can be a safe place for her?

Areas for Exploration

- How can I invite and engage at minimum Vali and Darci into counseling sessions, but the whole family if possible, in a way that all parties would be receptive to and feel safe to participate?

Suggested Strategies

- Discuss your role as a counselor in this case with Vali and Darci (when she called initially).
- Make clear what information you will keep confidential and what the limits of confidentiality are from the outset.
- Explain what information and how it will be used/shared if her family participates in counseling. Be sure to have signed consent to release information from all parties where information will be shared.
- Don't make promises you can't keep or expect Vali to automatically trust you – in fact, acknowledging that not trusting you right away is wise given you just met and her prior experiences. This can alleviate pressure for Vali to feel like she has to talk about things she may not desire or be ready to discuss. This can contribute to creating safety, show that you trust her judgment, and are willing to let her lead.
- Go slowly developing a good working relationship with Vali through joining, empathy, validation, reflection, and acknowledging her position and view.
- After Vali indicates her relationship with her mother, is particularly concerning and distressing to her, more than anything else, offer that counseling may be a place to work on that relationship.
- Explore with Vali the possibility of including Darci in counseling, including the pros and cons. Validate Vali's concerns as well as the benefits she can see.
- Verbalize understanding that both Vali and Darci are hesitant to participate in counseling, but both have a desire for the other to relate differently and improve their relationship.
- Acknowledge that it seems it may be as concerning to her mother, since she really wants things to be better for Vali, but doesn't know what else to do. If Vali is interested in inviting her mother to counseling, suggest Vali asks her mother to come to the next session with her, letting her know it would mean

a lot for her to be there and it could really help her to have her present. If she is uncomfortable with this, you can offer to call Darci.

- If Darci attends next session, reiterate your role, parameters around information sharing, and limits of confidentiality.
- Compliment Darci for attending to support her daughter, acknowledge how helpful that will be for Vali and understand how difficult this has been for her and you can see how much she cares for her daughter.
- Develop a good working relationship with Darci, understand her position, validate her concerns as a mother, and acknowledge social/political/cultural/familial factors influencing her concerns.
- Be sure to intervene to manage family conflicts and hostility. Maintain a neutral or multipartiality position. Since you have already been meeting with and joining with Vali, some unbalancing may be necessary to join with Darci (Minuchin & Fishman, 1981).
- Begin to work toward a relational and systemic definition of the problem where they find agreement (e.g., both would like to improve their relationship and find ways to express concerns in a way that will be well-received).
- If Darci refuses to attend, or Vali does not want her mother to participate, continue to work with Vali individually regarding her concerns with her mother and their relationship or on what she finds most concerning to her at the time.

BOX 14.2 WORKING WITH VALI

A Cultural Contextual Focus and Working with All Systems

Case Considerations and Areas for Exploration

- How is Vali's cultural context unique? What are the implied and overt messages, patterns of interaction, rules, coalitions, hierarchies, and cultural values of the multiple systems involved in Vali's life?
- Who am I in relation to this client, family, and society? How am I interacting with all of those person/systems? What are my assumptions, values, biases, and blindspots in this case? Whose story do I buy into? Whom am I aligned with? What direction am I taking? What questions am I asking or things I'm paying most attention to? How am I languaging my responses?
- What are the various systemic issues, participants, and context involved in this specific case where each member's behavior/responses make sense?

a e.g. Could Vali's anger toward her mother be an attempt to put distance in the relationship and have more independence?
b Could Darci's controlling behaviors be a reaction of fear and concern to the threats to her family's safety and her daughter's well-being?
c Could the family's handling of Vali be related to their social/political/cultural context, where government, society, and other professionals have reified their concerns?
d Could Vali's mood swings and conflicts with her family be a reaction to the violence and blame she experienced, but can't talk about, that may also be attempt to prove she is not a weak victim?
e Could the treatment and view of Vali by others stem from society's views on trauma, rape, abortion, and pathology?

- How can working with Vali and Darci (and hopefully other family members) to change their relationship lead to larger changes that might address other concerns such as moving past the trauma experienced, decrease mood swings and anger, expand Vali and Darci's systems of support?
- Are there ways to engage Vali and Darci in larger social/political/cultural changes?
- What are other possible resources for this family? Are there clubs or groups at the university where Vali would find support, camaraderie, or advocacy? Are there ways Darci can connect to the community in a way that will help her feel less fearful and safer?

Suggested Strategies

- Create a cultural genogram (Gilgun, n.d.; Hardy & Laszloffy, 1995) with Vali and Darci to map out cultural influences across time, account for various systems involved in the case and demonstrate the problem is not just within Vali.
- Use circular questioning (Selvini, Boscolo, Cecchin, & Prata, 1980; Penn, 1982) to draw out the relationship and process of interaction between people, which will reiterate a relational definition of the problem for all and help you understand Vali, Darci, and others' responses in their relational context, along with illuminating the patterns of interaction, rules, coalitions, hierarchies, and cultural values of the multiple systems involved in Vali's life.
- Develop with Vali and Darci new ways of relating to each other that they both are willing and able to engage in and lead toward their shared vision for an improved relationship that are not counter to their social/political/cultural/familial context.

Recommendations

It is common for family counselors to encounter involuntary clients in their clinical practice and this family-based cultural contextual approach offers the family counselor a systemic, ethical, and culturally sensitive way to engage with involuntary clients. When family counselors are able to understand the complex nature that makes a client involuntary, they are then able to begin working within the client's unique context. Family counselors must recognize and know how to work within the complex web of relationships they are a part of when working with involuntary clients. Working in this manner encourages willing participation in treatment and demonstrates honor, dignity, and respect all clients deserve. The family-based cultural contextual approach guides family counselors through working with involuntary clients, while also attending to the other systems involved in the client's life and treatment.

References

Anderson, H., & Gehart, D. (Eds.). (2007). *Collaborative therapy: Relationships and conversations that make a difference*. New York: Routledge.

Baker, K. A. (1999). The importance of cultural sensitivity and therapist self-awareness when working with mandatory clients. *Family Process*, 38(1), 57–67.

Bateson, G., Jackson, D., Haley, J., & Weakland, J. (1956). Toward a theory of schizophrenia. *Systems Research and Behavioral Science*, 1(4), 251–264. doi:10.1002/bs.3830010402.

Becvar, D. S., & Becvar, R. J. (2013). *Family therapy: A systemic integration* (8th ed.). New York: Pearson.

Becvar, R. J., Canfield, B. S., & Becvar, D. S. (1997). *Group work: Cybernetic, constructivist, and social constructionist perspectives*. Denver, CO: Love Publishing Company.

Boden, R. (n.d.). Culturally relevant supervisor: Ethical practice. Retrieved from www.supervisionceu.com/documents/courses/course_cr.pdf.

Brodsky, S. L. (2011). *Therapy with coerced and reluctant clients*. Washington, DC: American Psychological Association.

Boszormenyi-Nagy, I., & Framo, J. L. (Eds.). (1965). *Intensive family therapy: Theoretical and practical aspects*. New York: Harper & Row.

Corey, G. (2017). *Theory and practice of counseling and psychotherapy* (10th ed.). Belmont, CA: Brooks/Cole Cengage Learning.

Friedlander, M. L., Escudero, V., & Heatherington, L. (2006). *Therapeutic alliances with couples and families: An empirically informed guide to practice*. Washington, DC: American Psychological Association.

Gilgun, J. F. (n.d.). *Cultural genograms according to Hardy & Laszloffy*. Retrieved from www.slideshare.net/JaneGilgun/doing-a-cultural-genogram.

Haley, J. (1997). *Leaving home: The therapy of disturbed young people* (2nd ed.). Levittown, PA: Brunner/Mazel.

Hardy, K. V., & Laszloffy, T. A. (1995). The cultural genogram: Key to training culturally competent family therapists. *Journal of Marital and Family Therapy*, 21(3), 227–237.

Hubble, M. A., Duncan, B. L., & Miller, S. D. (Eds.). (1999). *The heart and soul of change: What works in therapy*. Washington, D. C.: American Psychological Association.

Lebow, J., & Black, D. A. (2012). Considerations in court-involved therapy with parents. *Journal of Child Custody*, 9, 11–38.
Lipchik, E. (2002). *Beyond technique in solution-focused therapy: Working with emotions and the therapeutic relationship*. New York: Guilford.
McGoldrick, M., & Hardy, K. V. (Eds.). (2008). *Re-visioning family therapy* (2nd ed.). New York: Guilford Press.
Micucci, J. A. (2009). *The adolescent in family therapy: Harnessing the power of relationships* (2nd ed.). New York: Guilford.
Minuchin, S., & Fishman, H. C. (1981). *Family therapy techniques*. Cambridge, MA: Harvard University Press.
Palazzoli, M. S., Boscolo, L., Cecchin, G., & Prata, G. (1978). *Paradox and counterparadox: A new model in the therapy of the family in schizophrenic transaction*. New York: Jason Aronson Inc.
Penn, P. (1982). Circular questioning. *Family Process*, 21(3), 267–280.
Ray, W. A. (2016, December 10). Accessing and utilizing relationship and contextual information in brief therapy. Retrieved from www.brieftherapyconference.com/download/CD06-Ray-MHEBT2016.ppt.
Rooney, R. H. (Ed.). (2009). *Strategies for work with involuntary clients* (2nd ed.). New York: Columbia University Press.
Selvini, M. P., Boscolo, L., Cecchin, G., & Prata, G. (1980). Hypothesizing - Circularity - Neutrality: Three guidelines for the conductor of the session. *Family Process*, 19(1), 3–12. doi:10.1111/j.1545–5300.1980.00003.x.
Snyder, C. M. J., & Anderson, S. A. (2009). An examination of mandated versus voluntary referral as a determinant of clinical outcome. *Journal of Marital and Family Therapy*, 35(3), 278–292.
Sotero, L., Cunha, D., da Silva, J. T., Escudero, V. and Relvas, A. P. (2016). Building alliances with (in)voluntary clients: A study focused on therapists' observable behaviors. *Family Process,* 56(4), 1–16. doi:10.1111/famp.12265.
Sotero, L., Major, S., Escudero, V. and Relvas, A. P. (2016). The therapeutic alliance with involuntary clients: How does it work? *Journal of Family Therapy, 38*, 36–58. doi:10.1111/1467-6427.12046.
Tavris, C. (1992). *The mismeasure of woman: Why women are not the better sex, the inferior sex or the opposite sex*. New York: Simon & Schuster.
Watzlawick, P., Weakland, J. H., & Fisch, R. (1974). *Change: Principles of problem formulation and problem resolution*. New York: W. W. Norton & Company.

Additional Resources

Haley, J. (1987a). *Problem-solving therapy* (2nd ed.). San Francisco: Jossey-Bass.
Haley, J. (1987b). Therapy: A new phenomenon. In J. Zeig (Ed.), *The evolution of psychotherapy* (pp. 17–31). New York: Brunner/Mazel.
Haley, J. (1992). Compulsory therapy for both client and therapist. In J. Carlson (Series Ed.), *Topics in family psychology and counseling, Vol. 1(2): Compulsory family therapy* (pp. 1–7). Rockville, MD: Aspen Publications.
Ivanoff, A., Blythe, B. J., & Tripodi, T. (1994). *Involuntary clients in social work practice*. New York: Walter de Gruyter.
Weakland, J. H., & Jordan, L. (1992). Working briefly with reluctant clients: Child protective services as an example. *Journal of Family Therapy*, 14, 231–254.

15

CULTURAL CONSIDERATIONS FOR COUNSELING AGING FAMILIES

Lori L. Soli and Susan J. Foster

Introduction

To live is to age. Inherently, families age and will face challenges related to hemostasis within this culture of aging. Changing roles and shifting expectations begin a journey of acculturation, resulting in the family's new reality. Though this chapter is positioned using a Westernized family, "the Rovers," all families will go through this process. Aging families, such as the Rovers, who get stuck in patterns of disequilibrium, often seek out solutions through counseling to their family's problems. Using the Integrated Experiential Approach, we provided the Rover family a safe place to explore collective empathy and awareness, craft a new family narrative, and re-rover their communication style (Soli & Foster, 2018a). Specific modalities, accompanied by traditional and adapted activities, were chosen to help meet the diverse needs of the Rovers and are illustrated using a case study approach.

This chapter explores the challenges that multigenerational families face in having one or more aging members, heretofore referred to as aging families. "Aging families" may be considered as a distinct group, in many aspects culturally different from others. According to the United Nations (2017), approximately 962 million people are 60 years of age or older in the world, accounting for 13% of the global population and is growing at a rate of 3% annually. This is unprecedented, as for the first time ever, there will be more older adults than children in the world, resulting in a new culture marked by longer life spans, new disease patterns, disability, increased costs associated with aging and care, and changing family structures and dynamics (Bailey & Johnson, 2016; National Institute on Aging, National Institutes of Health, & World Health Organization, 2018; Qualls & Williams 2013). On the upside, aging has taken on a vibrancy and hopeful tone also unprecedented in known history (Peluso, Watts, & Parsons, 2012). The new boom is the aging family defined by Johnston, Bailey, and Wilson (2014) as "any family system actively experiencing or planning for aging related changes" (p. 149). This family experience of switching roles and shifting familiar transactional patterns ushers in a new reality, a family culture; they become an *Aging Family*. Peluso et al. (2012) aptly highlight the rich possibilities and significant need for family therapists to better address the rapidly emerging needs of aging families.

As the traditional family unit becomes an aging family, significant changes occur, often without cognitive recognition of the acculturative process the family is immersed within. A disruption in family homeostasis occurs; within this new culture, role diffusion is likely. Readers will explore the culture of aging families and its challenges through the lens of the Rover family. While specifically exploring the Rover family's experience of an elder with Alzheimer's, given the universal characteristics of family units, the strategies offered are generalizable and can be modified to meet a spectrum of intercultural concerns aging families face.

The chapter positions Mr. Rover as the identified "symptom" within his Westernized family, however, the aging family is the identified client struggling with a developmentally necessary cultural shift that organically emerges in every aging family. Reflecting contemporary norms, the Rovers are a family of origin, union, and choice. Physical presence is not a qualifier to be "in the game"; all members are affected as the battle rages to regain the once known family homeostasis, now an illusion. Subsequently, the suggested strategies are mindfully designed to impact the aging family as a whole, whether conducted with individuals, groups, or the whole family.

Interventions

Experiential family therapy approaches are grounded in the notion that intellectualized logic takes a backseat to firsthand personal experiences and interactive processes, which when reflected upon, can produce new understanding, emotions, and behaviors (Bauman & Belous, 2016; Kolb, 1994; Smith, 1998; Whitaker & Bumberry, 1988). Incorporating active, multisensory techniques gives rise to an increased expression of affect, and greater perceptual flexibility while creating a heightened healthy interdependence is promoted (Jencius, 2017; Johnston et al, 2014). At its core, experiential counseling can be viewed as a vehicle which enables the client, in this case the family, to become the kind of person (in this case family) they want to *be*, rather than focusing on solving problems or symptom reduction. Grounded in diverse tenants from experiential family therapies, the Integrated Experiential Approach focuses on the possibilities and potential for the family to move toward valued living and aims to meet the complex and contextual needs of aging families.

While many have proffered integrative approaches to family therapy (Hassan, Jarrott, & O'Hora, 2014; Hawley & DeHaan, 1996), our approach is a consciously constructed blended application of several modalities designed with specifically experiential elements to address the challenges an aging family culture presents. A host of specific strategies located within four modalities, and holistically grounded in the Integrated Experiential Approach (Soli & Foster, 2018a) will be applied to address the presenting "problems" of family role diffusion and disruption. The approach is mindfully crafted to promote interfamily empathy, awareness, and communication while building new skills to consciously increase workable family transactions, adopt new roles and collectively move toward a more fluid family balance amidst their new cultural reality. The efficacy of the approach rests on the universal reality that within the aging family extant structures become extinct. The approach blends interventions to assist the family to decrease fusion with the obsolete structure, paralleling the families evolving, transformation which while developmentally unavoidable, is still existentially terribly hard.

The interventions (activities) employed in the case example are intentional, strategic reinventions of evidence-based practices and perspectives based on Design Thinking (Dalsgaard, 2014; Shute & Razzouk, 2012), Acceptance and Commitment Therapy [ACT] (Harris, 2008, 2009, 2018; Hayes, Strosahl, & Wilson, 2012), Narrative Therapy, Transformational Systemic Therapy (Satir, Banmen, Gerber, & Gomori, 1991), and Experiential Family Therapy (Mahrer, 1995; Whitaker & Bumberry, 1988). A brief introduction to each modality and proposed activities follows.

Design Thinking

While not necessarily a therapeutic modality, design thinking is an innovative approach built on the premise that all problems are ultimately resolved by stakeholders who collaboratively work to gain a shared understanding of the concern (Dalsgaard, 2014). From a family counseling perspective, this creates conversations based on "and" relationships, as opposed to "or" relationships. Further, design thinking can allow for the nurturing of a corpus of thoughts, feelings, and behaviors that lead to change in the wake of concern. Thus, the purpose of this modality is to assist families in developing empathy and understanding. In this chapter, design thinking is used to assist the aging family in developing awareness by building empathy around the identified problem. We will use an adaptation of the five stages of design thinking in an author-developed intervention called "Rock Solid" (Foster & Soli, 2018a).

The Satir Family Therapy Model

Self is the most important tool for change. The Satir Model of family therapy, developed by Virginia Satir, is a culturally relevant approach that focuses on the core belief that all individuals have internal resources and choices, which will ultimately bring transformational change within the individual, family and social systems (Satir et al., 1991). Germane to this approach is the notion that each individual within the system must connect with their core or essence. Only within this authentic identity and esteem can the individual move towards change. This awareness allows individuals to reframe problems as purposeful, with the recognition that the problem is really how we function and cope. Sculpting is often used to promote such awareness, as it provides a clear picture of what is happening in the family and how the family is reacting to it. In this chapter, we will use digital sculpting (Foster, 2018), a modern adaptation of family sculpting, as a tool to develop an understanding and communication of self, as it relates to being in an aging family.

Acceptance and Commitment Therapy (ACT)

ACT, a modality stated as an action verb, not initials, focuses on the premises that life brings pain, people can learn skills to handle painful feelings and thoughts effectively, and that clarifying what truly matters to an individual or group can inspire and motivate them toward life enriching goals and actions (Harris, 2009, p. 2). ACT can assist the aging family with experiencing its interactions in the present moment, decreasing experiential avoidance, and increasing experiential acceptance. In this chapter, ACT is used to help the aging family build understanding and communication and to help them develop new skills. ACT-based interventions employed will include values clarification, *Sky and Weather* metaphor, a variation of Harris The Folder, and skill-building activities based on the FEAR, DARE, acronyms (Harris, 2009; Hayes, 2005).

Narrative Therapy

Narrative Therapy rests on the premises that people have many interacting narratives (stories) which ground their sense of self, that current and past cultural discourse on power and identity influence presenting problems, and these problems are not restricted to nor located solely within clients. Centering on active engagement in re-storying narratives by re-considering, appreciating, and authoring their lives and relationships Narrative therapy provides avenues for the aging family to understand their current personal story better and offers meaning-making strategies to alter the trajectory of future life stories (Madigan, 2011; Noble & Jones, 2005; White & Epston, 1990). Narrative-based applications to promote understanding, communication, and new skills will be employed. Author-modified applications include creating a new lexicon of family role names which externalize the lived experiences of the family members by providing an alternative frame for the families "characters," Verb-ing Nouns – a tangible way to externalize and draw attention to old and new storylines, integrating old and new stories into digital sculpting, and narrating a unique life story via the Rover Game (Foster & Soli, 2018b).

Case Example

The "Rovers" are a family in the throes of living in the culture of an aging family, which is defined as *one who has a member or members experiencing age-related problems or challenges linked to the aging member is by nature a culture different than a family without*. The family is experiencing significant role diffusion, disequilibrium, and communication breakdowns. The Rover family has entered counseling at the request of Camilla, wife of the aging Penn Rover.

There are nine key players who emerge within the Rover family. **Penn Rover** has been very recently diagnosed with mild-mid stage Alzheimer's. He is a proud, down-to-earth, hardworking man who has enjoyed a lifelong career as a woodworker. **Camilla** has been Penn's wife for 40 years. She is a self-reliant, educated woman who embraces aging as an opportunity for continued growth. She has consistently enjoyed her professional career and travel. **Saphira** is Penn and Camilla's first-born daughter who self-identifies as having a "typical first-born" personality. She is divorced and has recently moved back into the family home to "take care of dad." **Molly**, daughter of Saphira and Dashe, is a grounded college student who has worked hard to overcome her own personal struggles. **Jeb** is Penn and Camilla's only son and middle child. He and his wife **Star** live close to the senior Rovers. They both have successful careers and have no children. **Ruby** is the youngest daughter who feels "stuck in the middle." **Dashe** is Saphira's ex-husband who remains close with the family. He does not live close to the Rovers. **Kas** is the openly bi-sexual longtime friend and confidant of Penn and Camilla.

The "Problem"

Consistent with the authors worldviews and the construct of their selected intervention approaches, "problems, are not problems." Families, however, present with a "problem" that needs to be fixed. We use the term "problem" to refer to the challenges, issues, concerns, and struggles the Rovers works through while acculturating as an aging family. Individually and collectively, the Rovers report feeling that deeply held values of who they *are* and togetherness has been fractured; members do not feel heard or valued. Problems have emerged for the Rovers as more and more members have switched "roles" either by choice or necessity, leaving the family in an unfamiliar state of disequilibrium and propelling all members into a perpetual game of "Familial Rover-ing." Role diffusion has resulted in diminished alliance, boundaries, problem solving, and ego states.

First Session

Camilla begins the session calmly discussing how much life has changed in the last year and is quickly interrupted by Saphira shouting "It's not *his* fault mom."

Penn, who is noticeably shaken by the exchange, keeps apologizing and repeating "I do not want to be a burden" and "I love you so much." Camilla and Molly exchange glances as if to communicate here we go again. Dashe tells Saphira to "Back off, it is nobody's fault, that's why we are here." Saphira interjects again stating "Everything would be just fine it you would just follow the plan." Jeb pipes in saying "The plan is not *Our* plan, it's *Your* plan and it's not working." Ruby smiles weakly at Jeb then looking at Saphira states "I just want things to be like they used to be where we were a team and work together, like dad always wanted, you know be *Us*." Saphira shoots the room a glare and under her breath she mumbles "You know that can't happen." Kas, to this point quietly observing, gets up and walks to position himself between Penn and Camilla then asks, "What do you want?" Star, re-crosses her legs, rolls her eyes, digs her fingers into Jeb's arm while fighting back tears.

Applying the Integrated Experiential Approach

Because of the complexity as evidenced in the snapshot, we employed the Integrated Experiential Approach (Soli & Foster, 2018a). While there is no "typical" aging family grappling with acculturation into, this approach allows for flexibility and meeting individual families where they are, thereby enabling counselors to help families articulate their particular "problems" within the greater cultural context. Within the Integrated Experiential Approach there are three stages: Awareness, Working, and Integration and Closure. Table 15.1 graphically represents how within each stage targeted, evidence-based interventions, both traditional and author-modified, are applied to the Rover family.

Intervention Strategy Application Stage 1: Awareness

Rocking the Status Quo with Design Thinking

Each Rover has a different idea of the "problem" and how it is affecting them. To begin the process of empathy and collective awareness, we employ a design thinking activity entitled "Rock Solid" (Foster & Soli, 2018a). The Rover family is given an asymmetrical rock and nine bendable straws. Without talking and using only the straws, the family is given one minute to move the rock across a table. After the task, we process the rock as a metaphor for the problem that brought them to counseling, what it was like to have a common problem, and the inability to communicate or have direction. Using the five stages of design thinking, we begin to develop a common language to define the problem. In the empathy stage, each family member is asked for their perspective on the problem and motivation for coming to counseling as a family. The family organically moves to a new stage of ideation and awareness, in which all opinions of the problem are viewed valuable. In the definition and prototype

TABLE 15.1 Integrated Experiential Approach Model

Stages	*Goal*	*Modality*	*Activities*
Stage 1: Awareness	Goal 1: Developing Empathy	Design thinking	Rock solid
		ACT	The Sky and The Weather Metaphor, I am having a thought that …
	Goal 2: Understanding and Communicating	Satir model/ Narrative	Digital sculpting
		ACT	The importance of importance
Stage 2: Working	Goal 1: Dealing with a New Reality	Narrative Therapy	Authentic self cards
	Goal 2: Building Skills	ACT	DARE-ing to Overcome FEAR
Stage 3: Integration and Closure	Goal 1: Integrating New Roles	Experiential Therapy	The Rover Game – Re-Rovering roles
		Narrative Therapy	Verb-ing nouns
		ACT/Narrative	Re-visiting importance and shining a light ahead
		Experiential Therapy	Rocking gratitude

phase, we theme the family dialog in such a way that the family now views the problem in more global, specifically fluid vs rigid terms. This new idea of the problem, role diffusion and communication impacting the family's acculturation into aging, is used as a basis for the experiential work in other stages of the counseling process.

Can the Sky Have a Thought That the Weather Sucks?

The Rovers each are fused to their thoughts and feelings about each other, their family roles, and the "problem." To provide the family a framework for extending one another empathy and encourage continual perspective taking, a platform for enhancing self-in-context reflection, we next introduce the ACT *Sky and Weather Metaphor* (review Medrano, 2017). Present the observing self as the sky, having ample space for *all* thoughts and feelings while remaining constant, neutral, and spacious. Thoughts and feelings are presented as the weather: unpredictable, sometimes stormy or hot and fierce, sometimes calm and mild. In parallel certainty to the sky's constancy, the weather *always* changes, and so do thoughts and feelings. Being nascent to exploring their often-difficult emergent thoughts and feelings in the current context, the metaphor's externalizing language promotes a shame-free internal alternative for the Rovers to move toward defusion. Next, we lead the Rovers through the ACT I'm Having a Thought That … technique (review Soli & Foster, 2018b) which equips them with another set of defusing tools. We continue to apply this technique in future sessions and encourage members apply it in and out of session to internally assist with creating a sky self, and externally to facilitate a communication.

Sculpting the Family Snapshot

As the family begins to develop new language to frame their problems in role diffusion and communication, we employ an adaptation of family sculpting called digital sculpting (Foster, 2018). The Rovers are asked to take a series of photos. In the first photo, each member is asked to quickly pose in response to the question, "How do you see yourself in your family?" Immediate reactions are captured in order to bring awareness to the members' current level of functioning in the family. In the second photo, each member is as to pose in response to "How would you want to be seen in your family?" Again, the goal was to capture their desire for change. Each set of photographs are arranged in before and after family portraits. The family reflected on individual and collective differences between the photos.

The Importance of Importance

What matters to me (what matters to the family) deep in my (our collective) heart and what do I (we) truly want? The Rovers must answer this complex question to move toward mindful action. We now engage the Rovers with clarifying values which leads to values-based behavior, which will contiguously serve to bring the Rovers closer to a new culturally relevant homeostasis. Have each member individually complete *A Quick Look at Your Values* worksheet from Harris (2018, pp. 23–24) using their favorite color, apply boundary-ing to ensure no one is required to share. Using a color that represents their family, have everyone complete the worksheet though the lens of what they believe the Rover family values are. Iterate that akin to all beliefs, family values are perceptual thus, not to perseverate over what other family members would say; this experience is individual. Have everyone list their top six Family Values on a separate paper and give to you. Process the activity encouraging members to "be the sky and the weather" and use I had a thought/feeling language. When the family returns to the next session, we created wall sized chart to share their collective listed values. We discuss similarities and differences highlighting there is no right or wrong values. We keep the chart posted during sessions and suggest the Rovers make their own notes on it as they are called to do so during sessions. We revisit the chart toward the end of counseling.

Case Study Intervention Strategy Application Stage 2: Working

Your Authentic Self Cards

Using the new awareness for self and change from Digital sculpting, each family member begins to develop their new narrative. Each member is given a card and asked to describe what their truest, genuine, most authentic self would be like we encourage using visuals as well as words and provide needed materials The Mind Reading Machine exercise from Harris (2009) can be used as a springboard for this activity. The cards will be saved and used in a later activity.

Pushing the Envelope

Since lives are made up of stories, within which our thoughts and feelings form, which swim in our heads perpetually like fish swim in the sea unaware they are swimming in water. Our next step with the Rovers is to facilitate a clearer understanding that the stories each tells themselves and the collective family story is not "the absolute truth" (Harris, 2008). This activity also provides a metaphor for discontinuing to push away unpleasantries, and practicing acceptance. We start by giving each Rover an empty, plain manila envelope and blank sheets of paper. As always, we have art materials available (e.g., markers, colored pencils, crayons). We have the Rovers each write down all the thoughts and feelings they are currently having about what is happening with them and with their family right now without editing. Allow 10 minutes and instruct when they are done they may personalize their envelopes as they wish. We now employ a modified version of the Pushing Away Paper Exercise (Harris, 2018, Appendix 6) titled Pushing the Envelope (Soli & Foster, 2018d) and have the Rovers form a circle with us located at the center. We proceed through the exercise narrating and modeling the activity from the middle. At the end, when all the envelopes are down, we ask the Rovers to look around the family circle and breathe in each of their family members for a full for 10 seconds, while thinking of at least one thing about each them for which they are grateful. We then pose the question "Are your gratitudes in your envelope?" Remind them that the story in their envelopes is a snapshot of a perspective caught in time, and not pure reality. They are always able to alter their focus, change the background, the narrative, and thus alter their new reality. We offer the thought that there is much more "truth" right in front of their eyes when they put the struggle down and contact the present moment.

DARE-ing to Overcome FEAR

We continue to work with the Rovers to find on identifying potential barriers to regaining a family equilibrium and putting their identified values into action. We introduce and discuss concepts of FEAR and DARE. To facilitate this, we use Harris (2018) FEAR 1–2 worksheets in session or as homework to assist the Rovers with identifying their barriers to values-based action (FEAR) and explore potentials for removing these (DARE).

Case Study Intervention Strategy Application Stage 3: Integration and Closure

The Rover Game – Role Re-Rovering

The Rover Game (Foster & Soli, 2018b) is a series of existential activities designed to facilitate an understanding of role diffusion and the struggle of working through and adapting to new family structures. Having increased collective empathy through previous activities, we employ *Role Re-Rovering* (Foster & Soli, 2018b) to integrate new family norms and continue arming the Rovers with skills to assess if their actions are workable and contribute to new cultural family values, meaning, and vitality, or contribute to the continued struggle and family suffering through fusion with an obsolete (extinct) family culture.

Introduce the concept that there are prototypical roles that each member of a family who is in the early stages of aging family acculturating might play. Read the Rover Role cards (Foster & Soli, 2018c) one by one and process which if any of the characteristics described resonate with how they perceive their former or current family role. As the Rovers identify with characteristics, approach this with levity and with the intent to illuminate the growth and progress already made. Next, bring out the Authentic Self cards created during the awareness stage and return to each person to review. Allow time to re-rover (i.e., revise, change, delete, add to) the Authentic Self cards as desired. To further illustrate and integrate communication skills, we will re-engage the family in the Rock Solid (Foster & Soli, 2018a) activity while mindfully embodying their re-rovered authentic self. Process the differences in how they confronted "the problem" in the initial experience and how they now confront the problem living within their more acculturated authentic collective self. Invite them to read their cards.

Verb-ing Nouns

As the Rover family strives to understand their newly emerging narrative related to the culture of aging, we led them in an activity entitled Verb-ing the Noun with the goal being continued externalization of the problem and engagement in a new storyline (Foster & Soli, 2018a). For instance, by bringing in parallels to the children's game "Red Rover," in which players build and eliminate alliances, the Rovers are able to process their own Rover-ing behavior. Then, using the Prototype Family Role Cards, the Rovers began to develop a collective verb-ing language that breathed life into their words and made them actionable (Foster & Soli, 2018d).We help the Rovers further apply this strategy to target their own and each other's accountability to move closer to their desired outcomes. For example, Camille might say to Ruby, "I am having a feeling you are Tanu-ing right now. What can I do to help you get closer to *You*," (referencing to Ruby's authentic self card).

Re-visiting Importance and Shining a Light Ahead

Using the Collective Family Values List created from the first values clarification activity, we create a one-page version and have the Rovers work through the list, prioritizing and personalizing what they believe to be their collective family priorities now. To further integrate new skills and establish workable boundaries, the Rovers collectively create a living family value statement using the steps from design thinking. To create a meaningful concrete post counseling action plan, we have each Rover complete the Harris (2018, p. 19) Willingness and Action Plan. After sharing and discussing, the Rovers will collectively create their own Family Willingness and Action Plan using the many tools and strategies they have learned throughout their Integrative Experiential counseling journey and implementing a consensus building model we have introduced such as Fists of Five or 1–2-4-All (Cohn, 2018). At this point where are entering closure and we to do a time capsule review all the stages they have gone through and progress gained through the approaches they have learn

Rocking Gratitude

As a final activity, we have the Rovers complete the Rocking Gratitude activity (Soli, 2018). The activity is a powerful verbal and physical reminder to each Rover that they not only matter, but they are an aging family, navigating their collective life without role diffusion, in homeostasis, an equipped to continue flexing with new family "problems" as they unfold.

By virtue of being a family and being alive, everyone must acculturate into being an aging family. All families will go through this process in their own ways, at their own pace and with their own processes. Family therapists are uniquely positioned to employ experiential activities to help meet the diverse needs of aging families in this process.

Conclusions and Recommendations

The authors worldview is predominantly a western lens, thus a western bias is implicit in the construction of the chapter itself. Readers are guided to alter activities to remain affirming of specific family customs and cultural contexts.

Pushing the Envelope

Before this activity carefully reviewed Harris (2018, Appendix 6) Pushing Away Paper Exercise because it is the basis for the activity. Be sure to spend time tailoring the language to fit the needs and goals of the specific family you are working with. Get clear with the activity so you do not need to read the script.

Cultural Sensitivity to Aging Family Members

Clients with age-related concerns (i.e., cognitive decline, mobility, hearing loss, sight loss) may be limited in their ability to fully participate in or may "fail" at some elements of the experiential activities. Counselors must be prepared for this possibility, actively model and create acceptance for and willingness to adapt and modify experiences to accommodate age-related limits and encourage in-the-moment processing. Part of the ongoing and overarching treatment plan should be a workable family plan to address current and emergent age-related concerns. Physical limitations of family members must be taken into consideration, however, changing the "rules" of the game should not be automatically altered by the counselor. Rather, help the family come up with a workable metaphor to adopt when someone in the family Does need an accommodation. Include an explanation that family rules are like the game rules; they simply exist and as long as the family accepts them as the status quo, they will comply. If accommodations "need" to be made, the family as a whole must decide and come to true (not "rovered") consensus on what to change.

Model Approach Language and Incorporate Metaphors

The Integrated Experiential Approach is laced with metaphors and new language. Integrate and model the language from the approaches as consistently as you can throughout sessions. This helps the family do the same and keeps the skill acquisition fresh.

Language for Homework

To reinforce the experiential and self-reflective elements of the model, we suggest using Harris' (2009) suggestion when assigning homework. First be sure to introduce homework in terms of trying an experiment to see what happens or doing something more about something else. Second, say something to the effect of let's make completing this a win-win, like we said practicing the new skills you are using both in sessions and through homework completion will really help you and your family work through the problems you have expressed. If you don't do this, I invite you to notice what stopped you. What thoughts came up that hooked you, what feelings came up that you struggled with, or what sorts of things did you do that got in your way?

Optional Session Assessment Tools

Using a session assessment tools can assist the counselor with better understanding how they are building alliances with the family. Using the SRS (Duncan 2012) is one way to do this. As well, since a continuous challenge in working with the Rover family is on the emotional struggles of regaining family equilibrium, the Struggling vs Opening Up Worksheet (Harris, 2018, p. 13) could be used at the end of each session to help each family member assess their in-session experiences while still in the moment. These could be dated and kept in the individuals manila envelope used in the Pushing the Envelope activity.

Space and Presence

A large space will be required for part of this intervention, which may necessitate careful planning for the counselor and family. When working with the family even before intake, recommend an early meeting with all family members present. You may want to schedule several sessions over a weekend to facilitate travel. If large-scale intervention is not possible physically, discuss the option for using telemental health capacities to "bring" all together into sessions when required.

Lenses

This chapter asks counselors to look through a very different "lens." Counselors are encouraged to take big leap of because the outcome of the activities is unknown. Confidence in group facilitation skills will be helpful. Testing of biases about aging is inherent in activities on the client and counselors/readers part. Modeling vulnerability and leaning into transparent conversation aligns with the Integrated Experiential Approach premise. In "Holding Space," the family counselor should be prepared for some powerful emotions to emerge and remain able to hold the space for each family client.

References

Bailey, W. A., & Gordon, S. R. (2016). Family caregiving amidst age-associated cognitive changes: Implications for practice and future generations. *Family Relations*, 65(1), 225–238. doi.org/10.1111/fare.12176.

Bauman, M. L., & Belous, C. K. (2016). Using symbolic-experiential family therapy to treat adjustment disorder: A case study. *American Journal of Family Therapy, 44*(5), 285–300. doi:10.1080/01926187.2016.1231599.

Cohn, M. (2018, April 24). Four quick ways to gain or assess team consensus. Retrieved from www.mountaingoatsoftware.com/blog/four-quick-ways-to-gain-or-assess-team-consensus.

Dalsgaard, P. (2014). Pragmatism and design thinking. *International Journal of Design,* 8(1), 143–155. Retrieved from www.ijdesign.org//IJDesign/article/1087/604.

Duncan, B. (2012). The partners for change outcome management system (PCOMS): The heart and soul of change project. *Canadian Psychology*, 53(2), 93–104. doi:10.1037/pst0000026.

Foster, S. (2018). Digital sculpting. Retrieved from https://integratedexperientialapproaches.wordpress.com/digital-sculpting/.

Foster, S. J., & Soli, L. L. (2018a). Rock Solid. Retrieved from https://integratedexperientialapproaches.wordpress.com/rock-solid/.

Foster, S. J., & Soli, L. L. (2018b). The Rover Game. Retrieved from https://integratedexperientialapproaches.wordpress.com/the-rover-game/.

Foster, S. J., & Soli, L. L. (2018c). Rover Role cards: Prototype family roles. Retrieved from https://integratedexperientialapproaches.wordpress.com/rover-role-cards-prototype-family-roles/.

Foster, S. J., & Soli, L. L. (2018d). Verb-ing the noun. Retrieved from https://integratedexperientialapproaches.wordpress.com/verb-ing-the-noun/.

Harris, R. (2008). *The happiness trap: How to stop struggling and start living*. Boston, MA: Trumpeter Books.

Harris, R. (2009). *ACT made simple*. Oakland, CA: New Harbinger.

Harris, R. (2018). Complete worksheets for Russ Harris books. Retrieved from www.actmindfully.com.au/wp-content/uploads/2018/06/2018_COMPLETE_WORKSHEETS_FOR_RUSS_HARRIS_BOOKS.pdf.

Hassan, K., Jarrott, S. E., & O'Hora, J. (2014). Therapists working in new and old ways: An integrative ecological framework for non-familial intergenerational relationships. *Australian and New Zealand Journal of Family Therapy*, 35, 207–222. doi:10.1002/anzf.1061.

Hawley, D. R., & DeHaan, L. (1996). Toward a definition of family resilience: Integrating life-span and family perspectives. *Family Process*, 35, 283–298. doi:10.1111/j. 1545–5300.1996.00283.x.

Hayes, S. C. (2005). *Get out of your mind and into your life: The new acceptance and commitment therapy*. Oakland, CA: New Harbinger.

Hayes, S. C., Strosahl, K. D., & Wilson, K. G. (2012). *Acceptance and commitment therapy: The process and practice of mindful change* (2nd ed.). New York:Guilford Press.

Jencius, M. (2017). Experiential family therapy. In J. Carlson & S. B. Dormer (Eds.), *The SAGE encyclopedia of marriage, family, and couples counseling* (pp. 578–581). Thousand Oaks, CA: Sage Publications.

Johnston, J., Bailey, W., & Wilson, G. (2014). Mechanisms for fostering multigenerational resilience. *Contemporary Family Therapy: An International Journal, 36*(1), 148–161. doi:10.1007/s10591-012-9222-6.

Kolb, D. A. (1984). *Experiential learning: Experience as the source of learning and development.* Englewood Cliffs, NJ: Prentice-Hall.

Madigan, S. (2011). *Narrative therapy*. Arlington, VA: American Psychological Association.

Mahrer, A. R. (1995). *The complete guide to experiential psychotherapy*. New York:John Wiley & Sons.

Medrano, M. (2017, July 24). The sky and the weather metaphor. Retrieved from www.counseling.org/news/aca-blogs/aca-member-blogs/aca-member-blogs/2017/07/24/the-sky-and-the-weather-metaphor.

National Institute on Aging, National Institutes of Health, & World Health Organization. (2018). Global health and aging. Retrieved from: www.who.int/ageing/publications/global_health.pdf.

Noble, A., & Jones, C. (2005). Benefits of narrative therapy: Holistic interventions at the end of life. *British Journal of Nursing*, 14(6), 330–333. doi:10.12968/bjon.2005.14.6.17802.

Peluso, P. R., Watts, R. E. E., & Parsons, M. (2012). *Changing aging, changing family therapy: Practicing with 21st century realities*. Hoboken, NJ: Taylor & Francis.

Qualls, S. H., & Williams, A. A. (2013). *Caregiver family therapy: Empowering families to meet the challenges of aging*. Washington, D.C: American Psychological Association.

Reiter, M. D. (2016). Solution-focused sculpting. *Journal of Systemic Therapies, 35*(3), 30–41. doi:101521jsyt201635330.

Satir, V., Banmen, J., Gerber, J., & Gomori, M. (1991). *The Satir model*. Palo Alto, CA: Science & Behavior Books.

Shute, V., & Razzouk, R. (2012). What is design thinking and why is it important? *Review of Educational Research, 82*(3), 330–348. doi:10.3102/0034654312457429.

Smith, G. L. (1998). The present state and future of symbolic- experiential family therapy: A post-modern analysis. *Contemporary Family Therapy*, 20(2), 147–161. doi:10.1023/A:1025073324868.

Soli, L.L. (2018). Rocking gratitude. Retrieved from https://integratedexperientialapproaches.wordpress.com/rocking-gratitude/.

Soli, L. L., & Foster, S. J. (2018a). Integrated Experiential Approach. Retrieved from https://integratedexperientialapproaches.wordpress.com.

Soli, L. L., & Foster, S. J. (2018b). I'm having a thought that … Retrieved from https://integratedexperientialapproaches.wordpress.com/im-having-a-thought-that/.

Soli, L. L., & Foster, S. J. (2018d). Pushing the envelope. https://integratedexperientialapproaches.wordpress.com/pushing-the-envelope/.

Soli, L. L. & Foster, S. J. (2019). Looking beyond the glass: Using the Johari window for (self) assessment in higher education. Retrieved from https://integratedexperientialapproaches.files.wordpress.com/2019/02/johari-hice-ppt.-handouts-lls1.2019.pdf.

United Nations. (2017). World population ageing. Retrieved from: www.un.org/en/development/desa/population/publications/pdf/ageing/WPA2017_Report.pdf.

Whitaker, C. A., & Bumberry, W. M. (1988). *Dancing with the family: A symbolic-experimental approach*. New York: Brunner/ Mazel.

White, M., & Epston, D. (1990). *Narrative means to therapeutic ends*. New York:W. W. Norton & Company.

Additional Resources

ACT

Gr8Talk [Screen name] (2012, February 14). Dr. Russ Harris Introduces ACT. Retrieved from www.youtube.com/watch?v=QS13jRcaufs

www.actmindfully.com.au

Alzheimer's

AARP.org/Disruptdementia

https://forum.alzheimers.org.uk/threads/carer-or-caregiver.14500/ www.alz.org/alzheimers_disease_stages_of_alzheimers.asp

Caregiver Information

www.healthinaging.org/resources/resource:caregiver-self-assessment. www.healthinaging.org
AARP.org/Preparetocare
AARP.org/Caregiving
Integrated experiential approaches
Our website

16

WORKING WITH TAIWAN COUPLES IN LIGHT OF CULTURE

A Case of Mother and Daughter-in-Law Relationship

Wentao Chao

Introduction

Before plunging into a discussion on culture, this author would like to make it clear that Taiwan families share a great deal of commonality in relational patterns with families in other societies, namely, most of the systemic theories could be applied to Taiwan families and provide helpful perspectives for counseling, if applied appropriately. The cultural framework proposed in this chapter does not intend to exclude other systemic perspectives, only to offer one more lens to help family counselors recognizing local relational patterns that could hardly be noticed otherwise.

Despite being a promising perspective, culture is not easy to grasp conceptually. First of all it covers a vast extensive range of ways of living, all the way from food to religions. Secondly, anthropologists, sociologists, and psychologists all define culture in different terms, making it even more complicated to focus. Thirdly, existed definitions of culture do not help much for clarifying relational patterns among family members, therefore are not very useful for a family counselor. All of the above leaves us no choice but to figure out a clinically useful definition of culture for ourselves.

The question is, could culture become a useful conceptual framework in understanding family relationship and interaction? To be specific, could the application of a cultural perspective helps a counselor understand Taiwan families better?

One domain this chapter would like to preclude exploring a possible application of culture in counseling is peculiar cultural practices, such as uxorilocal marriage (i.e., a man resides with his wife's family, and his children take the wife's family name). Although uxorilocal marriage does exist in Taiwan and it is intriguing, it is an unusual phenomenon, therefore not what this chapter aims to focus on. This chapter wants to explore common cultural beliefs or practices in Taiwan that seem to have an apparent impact on or even interference with family relationships, such as mother-in-law to couple relationship, or filial piety to parent–child relationship, phenomena that are prevalent and pivotal to Taiwan families.

A Definition of Culture for Family Counseling

To define culture that works for family counselors, this author proposed: culture defines, describes, and regulates socially approved "normal" and "appropriate" ways through which individuals develop themselves, satisfy their needs, and are expected to fulfill responsibilities and duties. In short, culture guides people through their lives for development and fulfilling expectations (Chao, 2016).

Once a culture has been established, it provides efficiency through predictability: things are relatively predictable if people in the same culture by and large follow the same relational norms. It even provides a sense of security: we feel safe with our loved ones if they behave predictably. Since people usually follow cultural norms without awareness, it gradually becomes an automatic process, and thus often reinforces itself. As a result, culture becomes dominant and entrenched, and individuals have less and less freedom in a cultural context.

Regarding culture, what concerns family counselors the most are first the means through which we strive for our well-being are essentially guided and also limited by our culture, with or without awareness. Second, our ways of coping with stresses and predicaments in life span are also deeply influenced by cultural context, even when they are not working. Third, cultural beliefs and customs possess a quality of self-reinforcement, therefore it takes effort, maybe from beyond the system, to break the self-reinforcing cycle.

Thus, one of the family counselor's tasks is to help families recognize how they are confined by their beliefs and customs rooted from culture, so they could respond to one another beyond their repetitive impasses. In fact, family counselors have been trained to dig into contexts for meanings underneath behaviors. Working with Taiwan families, sooner or later family counselors would come across beliefs and relational patterns that relate to culture, if they were not obscured by textbook theories. Since these cultural beliefs and customs usually stem from historical contexts and are shared by many local families, sensitivity to local culture definitely helps counselors further comprehend what is happening in the family.

For instance, relational duties and expectations are absolutely pivotal in Chinese families. People are expected to behave and interact with one another by relational structure, usually hierarchical, such as parent–child, more than by their needs. Obviously this could often result in disappointment and conflict. An adult son may feel suffocated by being obliged to obey his father's expectation for his decision, but simultaneously feels guilty if he rebels against his father's wish and feels ashamed by failing to fulfill filial piety. If a counselor works hard helping this man develop individuation without understanding and considering his cultural dilemma, the individuation process is not likely to work well for him.

Dilemmas of Applying Culture in Family Counseling

Plenty of existed literature has explored the role of culture in working with Chinese families. In a review this author categorized these publications into two groups: (1) Descriptions of characteristics in Chinese families, such as harmony emphasis, family cohesiveness, etc.; (2) Suggestion for culturally conformed intervention strategies, such as a therapist should demonstrate expertise and authority, respect hierarchy, set concrete and practical therapy goal, etc. (Chao, 2017).

One of the dilemmas of applying culture in family counseling is that, being knowledgeable about a culture doesn't guarantee success in counseling. When a counselor adopts a position of a "culture expert," he/she is prone to simplifying and stereotyping the family, which is obviously nontherapeutic. To enhance cultural sensitivity yet avoid stereotyping is the first challenge for family counselor.

The fact that a counselor is from the same culture doesn't guarantee sensitivity to the cultural impact on relational dynamics. People always take their own culture for granted, so they are blind to it. Family counselors from Taiwan also need, and particularly need, training for cultural sensitivity to Taiwan family cultural dynamics.

Many pertinent papers have suggested that counseling should conform to Chinese culture to maximize therapeutic effect with Chinese families, such as focusing on practical solutions, or avoiding open conflicts (Berg & Jaya, 1993; Ho, 1987; Hsu, 1995; Shon & Ja, 1982). Counseling strategies that correspond to culture may be easier for local families to comply, but there are times when counselors need to help families overcome restriction from culture and develop alternative way of relating, namely to challenge against instead of conforming to the culture. When to conform yet when to challenge – that is another dilemma.

One of the tricky challenges for counselors working with Taiwan families can be when theory contradicts cultural practice. One common conflict of such is the theory of differentiation of self vs. filial piety in parental relationship. Since filial piety plays such a significant role in Taiwan families, clients are often torn between desire for individuation and entangled feelings of shame and guilt. This contradiction presents a special challenge for family counselors in Taiwan, maybe in other Asian societies as well.

Counseling training programs both in USA and in Taiwan have been enhancing students' sensitivity to cultural diversity. This sensitivity to different ethnicities or to underprivileged populations helps counselors respect differences and practice social justice in counseling. Nevertheless this author considers sensitivity to cultural diversity is essentially different from study of a local culture. In Taiwan, the issue of culture in counseling has not much to do with ethnicity or underprivileged populations, but has more to do with traditional ways of interaction in relationship that shared by many local families yet often occurred unwittingly, to the degree people are collectively confined for their well-being.

Family counselors in Taiwan are mostly trained based on translated textbooks, so it is not surprising that they do not see cultural family dynamics just like their clients. It may be worth noting the distinction between cultural diversity and sensitivity to local relational patterns, and enhancing training accordingly for counselors working with Taiwan families.

For foreign counselors to become familiar with a culture, they need contact with it and to learn about it; nonetheless for counselors from Taiwan, it is probably the other way around: they need to distance themselves from this culture in which they have been embedded so deeply, to develop sensitivity and alternative perspectives, so they can begin to see the trace of culture in the families they work with.

Case Example

The following case is a combination of multiple clinical cases that the author worked with in Taiwan, to illustrate how culture can be incorporated into conceptualization in family counseling. For this purpose, only aspects relating to culture in the counseling process are presented here.

This was a couple in their 30s, with two daughters both going to preschool. The husband (let's call him Kevin) worked as an engineer, the wife, Jessie, housekeeping. They came for counseling because they had been in serious conflicts over almost all issues for several years, to the point of considering divorce when they came to see a marriage counselor.

One of the Jessie's complaints was about her mother-in-law. She claimed her m-i-l disdained her, criticizing her, and she felt stressed around her m-i-l. The husband refuted Jessie's complaints as nonsense, saying his mother didn't mean any harm in those situations, and suggested his wife should accommodate her m-i-l; after all, she was an elder.

There were many ways to help this couple: by strengthening the bounding between them, they could become better united and begin collaborating to work out the impact from mother-in-law. In this respect, traditional couple counseling that aimed at enhancing attachment and communication might work for this couple to a degree.

Individual counseling for Jessie might also help: if she could work on and gain self-esteem, Jessie might be able to cope better with her m-i-l without feeling overwhelmingly vulnerable, and hence transferring her resentment to her husband. Moreover, if Jessie could further differentiate herself from her family of origin, she might be more capable of maintaining a better boundary between herself and her mother-in-law, which would definitely reduce her distress.

However, the issue of mother-in-law is so prevalent in Taiwan it was obviously not just happening in this marriage, and it seemed to relate to some cultural dynamics. First, the relationship between daughter and mother-in-law was not really equal (Chao, 2016), it was considered as a "quasi-parent-daughter" relationship, in which a m-i-l usually expected her d-i-l to obey like a daughter. Vice versa, a daughter-in-law would also expect her m-i-l to treat her like a real daughter, and inevitably found a discrepancy between her expected way and how her m-i-l actually treated her (Kung, 2001). So here we had two women trying hard to behave like a family, yet were sensitive to whether the other party intended the same. All of the above gave the already difficult relationship between mother and daughter-in-law even more weight to deal with.

Like many wives stuck in this situation, Jessie was disappointed for the relationship didn't go well with her m-i-l, and yet she couldn't speak for herself because she hadn't had an "insider" position in her in-law family (Kung, 2001), therefore she was seriously frustrated, depressed, and resentful.

In a traditionally hierarchical relationship between daughter and mother-in-law, it is difficult for a daughter-in-law to speak for herself against the elders in her in-law family. A daughter-in-law often needs to work hard to earn her "membership" in her in-law family. This usually means to be a strong ally and a diligent domestic helper to her m-i-l. When a daughter-in-law could not perceive enough goodwill from her m-i-l to support her endeavor, she would be frustrated and discouraged.

In view of the above cultural dynamics, the counselor helped Jessie reflect and renegotiate her expectations on the relationship with her m-i-l. How did she see the role of a daughter-in-law? Had she worked too hard to please her in-laws in order to melt into the family? Did she know how to relate to her m-i-l in less sensitive aspects of life? How had/could her husband help(ed) her establishing a functional relationship with her m-i-l? After all, he had known his mom much longer than Jessie.

The above conversations were designed to expand Jessie's repertoire from the traditional in-law relationship, and figure out alternative ways of relating to each other. This process also involved Kevin the husband, so the couple relationship could also be enhanced along the process.

On the other hand, a mother-in-law is often extremely sensitive about whether her son retains filial piety after marriage to his wife. If she perceived any change of attitude, she would feel insecure because her well-being for the rest of her life might depend on the degree of her son's filial piety toward her, or at least her expectations. Since she can't be mad at her son to win back his filial piety, she usually blames her daughter-in-law for her son's disloyalty, and becomes resentful against her d-i-l. In other words, when in-law relationships goes sour, there might be insecurity behind resentment and pickiness of the mother-in-law.

A mother-in-law might also feel ambivalent toward her daughter-in-law. First of all this relationship is likely to elicit her own experience as a daughter-in-law in the past, which was often bitter or even of suffering in the early days. Now as a mother-in-law she needs to adjust to a new generational standard of mother and daughter-in-law relationship, and at the same time digest her own past traumatic experiences in the in-law relationship. Moreover, when she chats about this in-law relationship with her female friends, many of whom are also mothers-in-law themselves, she might get all kinds of advice for tackling her daughter-in-law. All these concerns and ambivalence make this in-law relationship even more delicate to manage.

Regarding the insecurity of a mother-in-law, it was crucial for the husband to reassure his mother of his filial piety, so his mom didn't have to worry about losing her son to her d-i-l. Unfortunately, most Taiwan husbands do not realize their crucial role in the mother and daughter-in-law conflicts, and often try to persuade their wives to accommodate the mother, or explain for his wife to his mother, and end up inevitably upsetting both women, and become helpless and withdrawn from this situation, leaving the two women to fall into further entanglement. Namely, if a husband couldn't see his role in a daughter and mother-in-law relationship, and accordingly provide timely reassurance, he could worsen the conflict despite his desire to help.

With the above perspectives in mind, the counselor asked Kevin whether he could appreciate his wife's distress and his mother's insecurity. He promptly replied that he could, saying he saw how stressful Jessie had been, but it didn't occur to him that his mother could feel insecure. The counselor responded that he wouldn't know, then invited the husband to consider if it's possible based on his knowledge of his mom. He nodded, saying it's possible. The counselor then invited him to explore possible ways to alleviate his mother's insecurity. The husband thought for a while, and said there were things he could do that would help. At this point, Jessie looked at Kevin nodding.

The counselor further explored what Kevin could do to make Jessie feel supported, because what a distressed wife needed the most was not a benevolent mother-in-law but a supportive husband. Jessie kept nodding to agree with this statement. Kevin turned to look at Jessie for a few seconds, then decided to ask her "What can I do to make you feel supported when things didn't go well with mom?" When Jessie was talking to her husband, the bitterness on her eyebrows seemed to be melting.

Kevin disclosed that he felt quite relieved after figuring out concrete actions he could do to mitigate the conflict between the two women he cared deeply, because the conflict had been bothering him for a while. Now in counseling he demonstrated remarkable willingness to help to dissolve the sorrow of his wife. Feeling that he could be helpful seemed to empower him, and being able to lessen Jessie's distress seemed to further motivate him to step out and take actions.

Jessie was pleased to see Kevin move from withdrawal and begin to take action that really helped. Once she began to feel Kevin's support, she became less vulnerable and reactive to her mother-in-law, and therefore was less disturbed. Although this couple still had many issues to argue about, in-law relationship was less mentioned in their bickering.

A Step Further: Mother-in-Law Joined Couple Counseling

Like most couple counselors, this author usually focuses his work with couples on the marital relationship. It never occurred to him to invite a mother-in-law to join couple counseling.

Nonetheless he did come across cases in which parents worried about their adult children's marriage and came to counseling with the couples. When that happened, he briefly talked to the parents to understand their worries, and left them outside the counseling room when interviewing couples because he believed couple counseling was supposed to strengthen the relationship between the couple, whereas parents' interference could only jeopardize the relationship between the couple and the intergenerational boundary.

However, Taiwan parents are concerned about their child's marriage as much as, or even more so, than their own marriage, and they sometimes do get involved without hesitation. Namely, these parents might have been meddling in their child's marriage no matter whether the counselor included them in couple counseling or not. So this author figures: is it possible to include mother- or father-in-law in a couple counseling session? Would it be helpful to do so? How could it be processed in ways that benefit all parties?

This author decided to explore this possibility. The following is a session in fiction based on the author's clinical experience of how the clients would respond in the pertinent context. First, this counselor decided to expand the couple's perspective to their mother's experience. He asked the couple if the mother knew that they had been bickering. Did she worry about their relationship? What did she do when she was worried?

The couple didn't have an answer for most of the above inquiries. They suspected that mother did worry about them, because she kept suggesting the couple come over to her place more frequently than earlier, and said she would like to see her granddaughters more often.

Now the couple seemed to realize their marriage had affected their mother in some degree, then the counselor explored with the couple whether their mother had also influenced their marital relationship. Jessie immediately confirmed, said she was very upset by Kevin's response when she mentioned her distress from her mother-in-law. When Kevin tried to explain that the reality actually didn't happen as per Jessie's exaggerated description, the counselor reminded him to find ways to support his wife, because she needed her husband the most when she was in distress. Kevin promptly shifted from explaining to accommodating

Jessie's complaint by listening attentively. When Jessie seemed to regain her composure, the counselor indicated that, if Jessie had been influenced by her mother-in-law, so Kevin must have been.

Then the counselor further explored with the couple: might their mother also feel distressed by her relationship with daughter-in-law? Was it possible that she wanted to establish a good relationship with her daughter-in-law, but didn't know how to approach? Both Kevin and Jessie confessed that they had never thought about these, and both agreed that it was likely so.

So the counselor began to explore the possibility for the couple to check with their mother on those suspicions. Both looked disinclined, feeling it would be awkward to talk about this with mom. When the counselor proposed to invite mother to join counseling for a session to have a conversation, both doubted that mother would ever come. The counselor agreed it was unusual to have this conversation if they were not used to disclosing their worries and concerns to one another at home.

It could be awkward at the beginning, but it might be meaningful for everyone involved.

In the next session, Kevin's mother, Carol, showed up with the couple for counseling. It was quite a surprise for the counselor, so he began the session by inquiring how Carol was invited and how she decided to join this session. Carol explained she didn't understand what counseling was and how it worked, but she had had a conversation days before with her son, and he had told her that he had been seeing a couple counselor with his wife for a while. Carol said she knew all along that the young couple had been bickering from time to time, but she had no idea how serious it was. What surprised her even more was her son told her that part of the bickering had to do with her.

The counselor asked Carol how she felt about this news. Carol said she absolutely wanted their marriage to be happier, but she thought it should be their own business so she had never intervened, therefore when her son told her that she was involved in their conflict, she was confused and clueless.

The counselor invited Kevin to help explain to Carol about her involvement. Kevin spoke to Carol in prudence: Jessie was a bit sensitive to her attitude toward Jessie, and became burdened in the relationship with her. Carol turned to look at Jessie, which seemed to make Jessie a bit uneasy. The counselor said that he knew Jessie had been trying to be part of this family, and asked Jessie if she would like Carol to help her with that. Jessie confirmed she would very much need Carol's help because she could not be sure how to respond to Carol's suggestions sometimes, worrying Carol might be upset if she had her ways, such as in parenting. Carol responded to Jessie that she only meant to provide her experience and help, but it was up to her to raise her children. Carol's tone sounded benevolent, which seemed to be a comfort to Jessie to a degree.

Then the counselor asked Carol how she liked her two granddaughters. Carol looked cheerful immediately, said the two girls were adorable, and she enjoyed the time with them. Kevin proposed to Jessie that maybe they should manage to visit Carol more often, because the girls loved to visit grandma too. This proposal would have imposed pressure on Jessie; nonetheless, Jessie seemed to be OK with it this time. She smiled when listening to her husband's proposal.

Carol only came for one session. She declined coming to counseling again when the counselor checked with her before the session ended. She said it was up to the young couple to work on their relationship; nevertheless she would be open to what they needed to tell her when they had something to tell her. The counselor expressed his appreciation of Carol's coming to help her son and daughter-in-law, and praised her wisdom to respect the boundary of the young couple.

The Following Sessions with the Couple

In the next session, the counselor inquired the couple, how was their experience in the previous session with Carol. Jessie disclosed she was nervous when she heard Kevin had told Carol about their conflicts, but she was glad that he checked with her before inviting Carol to join the session. Jessie said she struggled for this invitation, and then decided to let Carol came, because Carol had been involving anyway, might as well having a chance to hear what she had to say.

Kevin said he was uneasy to have his mother join the session too, but after he talked to Carol about his bickering with Jessie, Carol's response surprised him. She said she had been worrying about their marriage, but she didn't really know how to help so she had been keeping silent. The sanity in Carol's tone gave Kevin hope. He thought it might be helpful if the three could sit down and talk. But he reckoned they would need a helper when this conversation took place, so inviting Carol to counseling became the most sensible move to make. Then Kevin mentioned that Jessie didn't respond positively to this idea in the beginning, and he didn't want to push her for it too. He was once again surprised when Jessie brought up a few days later that she was ready to have Carol join the counseling.

Kevin explained he was excited about Jessie's change, but then worrying that Carol would not accept this idea easily. So he waited for a chance in which he had time alone with Carol, and carefully revealed Jessie's distress in relationship with Carol. Kevin declared this kind of conversation never occurred before between him and his mom, but it turned out to be surprisingly enjoyable. In that conversation, Carol expressed her surprise about Jessie's distress, and claimed she would not wish Jessie to suffer because of her. Relieved to hear that, Kevin invited Carol to join the counseling for once, so Jessie could hear Carol's good wish. Carol didn't understand why Jessie and her could not have this conversation at home. Kevin explained to her Jessie could feel a bit daunted by confronting her mother-in-law, she might need some help to speak up to her. Under Kevin's sincere invitation, Carol promised to come to counseling once to help her son and daughter-in-law's marriage.

Jessie was intimidated when Carol stared at her at some point in the session. She felt cornered and quite restless. She also remembered hearing Carol say that Carol would respect her ways of parenting. Although she wasn't sure if she could believe Carol 100%, she felt somewhat relieved. Despite Jessie could not remember many details in the conversation, she experienced a warm and kind quality in the relationship with Carol, which was new to her.

Kevin confessed he was also daunted when he had to explain to Carol that Jessie was sensitive and burned in the relationship with Carol. He wasn't sure how Carol would react to that. Fortunately Carol soon expressed her willingness to help lessen Jessie's distress, which seemed to turn things around. Kevin appreciated the counselor mentioned the granddaughters. He saw how cheerful and benevolent Carol instantly became when talking about her two angels. He considered that a smart move in making the conversation friendly.

After the joint session, Jessie said she still felt somewhat uneasy in setting boundaries between her and her mother-in-law over various issues, nonetheless in a much less degree. She didn't consider Carol picking on her on purpose any more, and she didn't feel as much distressed when visiting Carol's place on holiday.

Kevin reported that their bickering had apparently reduced, though there were still many other things to argue about. At least now he felt much relief that these two women basically respected each other, and both tried to maintain a harmonious relationship. In fact, after this process, Kevin found himself became closer to his mom. He felt easier to share things with her. That was an unexpected bonus.

Reflections on Including Mother-in-Law in Couple Counseling

To include mother-in-law in a session is definitely unusual in couple counseling. This author decided to explore this possibility in this chapter, hopefully to inspire more alternatives and reflections for a feasible counseling maneuver.

Although the joint session part of the case is fictional, it is also reasonably possible to really occur in counseling. Furthermore, what the counselor does in the session is also feasible. Therefore, after the above exploration, this author is convinced that it is a feasible move in counseling for a Taiwan couple.

In fact, it is the most logical consequential move after conceptualizing the couple's distress in the cultural perspective. The wife's mother-in-law had been involved in their marital relationship, with or without the mother-in-law's active participation. Since the impact had been happening, it is actually unreasonable not to incorporate it into conceptualization.

The merits of including mother-in-law in couple counseling, however, are multiple. Firstly, it ensures and strengthens the husband's pivotal role to be the bridge between his wife and his mom. Through the bridging process, the likely conflict between the two women gets to transform into a matter of balance among the three, with the husband in between lubricating the relationship. Apparently it is much more promising to balance this delicate in-law relationship with the husband/son's maneuver.

Secondly, it creates an opportunity for the daughter-in-law to have a direct conversation with her mother-in-law, instead of speculation and suspicion. Once they get to talk face to face, things are usually much easier. However, a daughter-in-law doesn't have an ethical position or chance to speak up to her mother-in-law, making this conversation difficult to bring about. This is exactly what counseling can offer for a daughter-in-law and her daunted husband.

Thirdly, this process helps a daughter-in-law begin to be aware of her mother-in-law's position, so she doesn't see her mother-in-law as a perpetrator and herself as a victim. Through a series of explorative inquiries, a daughter-in-law will be able to understand and empathize with her mother-in-law, and thus develop a humane relationship accordingly.

Fourthly, this process also helps the husband reconnect with his mother. Despite his relationship with his mom before, this task urges him to open himself to his mother on his marital challenges, and gives mother a chance to understand her adult son's life distress. If lucky, both mother and son will find this process facilitates their relationship.

Nevertheless it is only one option to invite mother-in-law to join the couple counseling session. There are always many means to achieve the therapeutic result, including not inviting mother-in-law to join the session. And of course it is always subject to the case to decide if it is appropriate or beneficial to include in-laws into a work of marital relationship.

Conclusions and Recommendations

This chapter intended to explore the possibility of applying culture as a conceptual framework in working with Taiwan families. This author argued for the need of defining a focus of culture that works for family counselors, and proposed one in this chapter. Then through a literature review he highlighted some possible challenges and dilemmas when applying culture in family counseling practice.

Then he presented a case to illustrate how culture can be incorporated into the counseling process with a Taiwan couple, followed by discussions and reflections on the merits of applying culture and other possible options to work with this case. The process of the case was presented in detail, so readers can really see how it proceeded and reflect on or criticize it.

The ways of conceptualizing culture in the case, and the counselor's specific maneuvers of working with the couple in this case, are merely one example of practice. This author doesn't mean to imply it is the only way or a better way, but only an alternative way. Hopefully it can inspire or expand other counselors in their own works.

References

Berg, I. K., & Jaya, A. (1993). Different and same: Family therapy with Asian-American families. *Journal of Marital and Family Therapy*, 19(1), 31–38.

Chao, Wentao (2017). Application of local cultures in family therapy: Literature review and reflections on practice. In P. H. Chen (Ed.), *Multi-cultural counseling in Taiwan* (chapter 10). Taipei: Psychological Publishing Co.

Chao, Wentao, Hsu, Junfong, Chang, Chishuang, Hus, Lai, Hsieh, Yifang, Lee, Juyu, & Lu, Buoje (2016). *The assessment and repair of family relationship in Chinese contexts: Seven stories of Taiwan families*. Taipei: Living Psychology.

Ho, M.K. (1987). *Family therapy with ethnic minorities*. Thousand Oaks, CA: Sage.

Kung, Hsiang-Ming (2001). Who is one of our own? The in-group/out-group effect on the relationship between mother- and daughter-in-law. *Indigenous Psychological Research in Chinese Societies*, 16, 43–87.

Hsu, J. (1995). Family therapy for the Chinese: Problems and strategies. In T.Y. Lin, W.S. Tseng, & E.K. Yeh (Eds.), *Chinese societies and mental health*. Hong Kong: Oxford University Press.

Shon, S. P., & Ja, D. Y. (1982). Asian families. In M. McGoldrick, J. K. Pearce, & J. Giordano (Eds.), *Ethnicity and family therapy*. New York: Guilford Press.

Additional Resources

Chao, Wentao (2011). Review and reflections on 40 years of family therapy development in Taiwan. *Journal of Family Therapy*, 33(4), 415–428.

Chao, Wentao (2018). The dialectical complementarity of East and West in me: Reflections of a family therapist practicing over 20 years in Taipei. *Asian Journal of Family Therapy*, 2(1), 11–24.

Sim, T., Fang, X.Y., Chan, S., Loy, J. T. C., Sng, S., Lo, R., Chao, W.T., & Singh, R. (2017). Co-constructing family therapy in the Asian Chinese family diasporas of mainland China, Malaysia, Macau, Singapore and Taiwan. *Journal of Family Therapy*, 39(2), 131–150.

17

FAMILY SYSTEMS THERAPIES WITH APPALACHIAN FAMILIES

Jason P. Austin, Benjamin J. Evans, and Ruoxi Chen

Introduction

Being culturally competent in the conceptualization and practice of family therapy entails more than reading textbooks, attending workshops, and participating in diversity seminars. Every individual, couple, and family are influenced by cultural values embodied in their geographical region. Family systems therapies have provided therapists with principles for approaching and situating oneself as a cultural outsider with diverse families. This chapter applies these principles to people residing in the Appalachia region of the United States, a geographical region spanning 205,000 miles across 13 states. Moreover, we discuss four unique cultural traits of the Appalachian people – family unity over personal progress, Appalachian personalism, distrust of outsiders, and fatalism – and family systems therapies principles using a case example of Cole and his family. Just like working with members of minority cultures, working with variations of the dominant culture involves cultural sensitivity during the joining, assessment, and intervention therapeutic stages.

Working with culturally diverse families can be a rewarding experience for family counselors as it challenges us to become more aware of our own implicit values as well as the those of our clients. Because our "epistemology leads to a particular way of arranging observed data" (Keeney, 1979, p. 118), we need to have at least a rudimentary understanding of that culture to work effectively with clients of a given culture.

Appalachians, often referred to as "an invisible minority" (Hayden, 2004; Russ, 2010), have often been overlooked (Gollnick & Chinn, 1998; Keller & Helton, 2010) in relevant cultural and diversity discussions. Despite being predominately White, Appalachians have a unique cultural identity central to their geographical location that must be considered in the context of treatment (Foster, 1988; Keefe, 1988, 2000). Moreover, Appalachian families have historically been characterized in pejorative terms (e.g., "hillbilly," "redneck," "mountain folk," "moonshiners," "inbred") and perceived as poorly educated individuals living in poverty and largely failing to contribute to our social condition (Foster & Hummel, 1997; Keefe & Greene, 2005). For family counselors working with Appalachian clients, it is extremely important that they are well informed of the unique cultural values often espoused by families living in this geographical region. The purpose of our chapter is to provide family counselors with a) a geographical and historical context of the Appalachia region, b) an overview of family systems theory as relevant to working with this population, and c) specific, culturally sensitive family therapy techniques via a case example.

A Brief Introduction to Appalachia

When thinking of Appalachia, most may only consider states containing parts of the Appalachian Mountains such as Kentucky, North Carolina, Tennessee, West Virginia, and Virginia. But Appalachia encompasses 420 counties sprawling 205,000 square miles across 13 states ranging as far south as Mississippi to as far north as New York and housing approximately 25.4 million people (Keller & Helton, 2010; Pollard & Jacobsen, 2017). Of the 420 counties comprising Appalachia, 67% are considered rural as compared with 21% of all US counties; 42% of Appalachians are rural as compared to 20% of the US population (Poole, et al., 2015). As such, many family counselors treating clients in Mississippi and/or New York may not realize that they are working with Appalachians. Furthermore, the fact these areas are culturally and contextually different from one another highlights the richness of the Appalachian regions' diversity.

Although currently 82.5% of the Appalachian population are White Non-Hispanic, the migration of racially and ethnic diverse minorities – such as African-Americans (9.4%), Hispanic Americans (4.6%), and many others (3.5%) – are increasing at higher percentages than national averages (Pollard & Jacobsen, 2011, 2017). Since the 1960s, Appalachia's poverty rate has been cut in half from 31% to 17.2% today, largely through the investment of public funds, although still above the national poverty rate of 15.6%. Appalachian per capita income is 81% of US per capita income, an increase from 74% in 1960. Appalachian educational attainment is also growing with 21.3% of adults age 25 years and older being college graduates, a figure that topped 5% in 1960. Furthermore, investment in Appalachian highway and road infrastructure has reduced the geographic isolation in the region while increasing commerce and economic opportunity. While Appalachia still lags behind the rest of the US in workforce participation, per capita income, housing quality, and health, the region has overall improved reflecting a positive direction of community development (Appalachian Regional Commission, n.d.; Pollard & Jacobsen, 2017; Poole et al., 2015).

Despite the improvements, Appalachians continue to experience hardship due to lack of available resources and geographic isolation in some regions. These hardships compound for Appalachians living in rural areas (Jackson et al., 2007) as they are disproportionately affected by heavier healthcare costs, less coverage, and higher access disparities than the rest of the US. For instance, Appalachians are at higher risk for substance abuse and mental health problems (Zhang et al., 2008), hospitalization (Hendryx, Ahern, & Nurkiewicz, 2007), heart disease (Hendryx & Zullig, 2009), and kidney disease (Hendryx, 2009).

Furthermore, rural Appalachians may not have access to appropriate mental health resources with 69% of nonmetropolitan Appalachian counties designated a mental health professional shortage area (Hendryx, 2008). Due to such lack of resources, as well as other social, economic, and regional barriers (Jackson, et al., 2007), Appalachian parents are more likely to seek treatment from school services and medical professionals long before seeking help from family counselors (Gore, Sheppard, Waters, Jackson, & Brubaker, 2016; Polaha, Dalton, & Allen, 2011).

Cybernetics, Family Systems Theory, and Family Therapy

Family therapy approaches, underlined by cybernetics and family systems theory, are highly recommended for working with Appalachian clients (Cole, 1988; Helton, 1995; Lemon, Newfield, & Dobbins, 1993). In particular, family systems based-approaches – such as structural therapy (Minuchin, 1974), MRI brief therapy (Watzlawick, Weakland, & Fisch, 1974), and strategic therapy (Haley, 1987) – seem to present a particular good fit in working with Appalachian families. Overall, these approaches tend to highlight the importance of observer imposed punctuation of events, therapists' role in the system, behavior as communication, interpersonal relationships instead of psychopathology, a focus on interactional patterns, context including the wider social unit, and a focus on changing behaviors instead of cognition (Watzlawick, Bavelas, & Jackson, 1967; Liddle, 1983; Keeney & Ross, 1985).

Structural family therapy assesses family functioning by exploring how families' boundaries, hierarchies, and subsystems are upholding problematic behaviors. Focusing on the present, structural family therapists do not explore extensive personal histories, and do not punctuate families as dysfunctional. Instead, they work with families to change how they relate to one another by challenging problematic hierarchies, highlighting covert coalitions, and restructuring misaligned boundaries (Gehart, 2014; Minuchin, 1974).

MRI brief therapy (Watzlawick et al., 1974) and strategic family therapy (Haley, 1987) both conceptualize problematic behaviors as "part of the interactional sequence of behaviors that have emerged through repeated exchanges, with no one person to blame" (Gehart, 2014, p. 64). MRI brief therapists focus on interrupting attempted solutions – or "more of the same" responses that through repetition uphold the symptomatic behavior – and metacommunication – or both the report (content) and command (nonverbal behavior) of interpersonal communication. Strategic family therapists often focus on the family's stage of life characterizing problems as "getting stuck" and not transitioning to the next phase (e.g., parents treating their son as a child instead of granting more autonomy respecting his developmental needs). Both approaches focus on the resolution of the presenting problem by interrupting problematic interactional patterns. MRI often uses reframing, prescribing the symptom, and restraining client progress while strategic therapists solely use directives (Gehart, 2014; Haley, 1987; Watzlawick et al., 1974).

Case Example

Appalachians share many cultural traits with rural southern culture (Denham, 2016; Duncan, 2001; Keefe & Greene, 2005). However, these cultural traits can be difficult to operationalize as "culture can be slippery and articulating what is meant by Appalachian can be a difficult task" (Denham, 2016, p. 97), creating a challenge for family counselors working with these families in culturally sensitive ways. Using a case example, we will now offer concrete examples of therapeutic interventions with Appalachian families, highlighting four salient traits of Appalachian culture we find important in the therapeutic process. At the same time, the cultural traits discussed here are not an exhaustive representation of Appalachian families and may not apply to all Appalachian clients, or even to the same degree.

Cole,[1] a 16-year old Caucasian male, lives in rural Appalachian with his father, Teddy, a divorced factory worker out of work due to traumatic brain injury from a car accident several years earlier, and reports having close ties to extended family, specifically an uncle and paternal grandparents. Teddy lived in a government subsidized local apartment complex with Cole and both report many of the complex's residents being involved in using and selling drugs. Cole often stole Teddy's prescribed medications for chronic pain and frequently traded them for other drugs with those residents.

Cole's paternal grandparents lived with an uncle, Sam, whom Cole reported being close to and is also his grandparents' favorite grandchild. Sam's home could best be described as the family home and was in a rural, wooded area on a large plot of land. Cole had his own room prepared where he could stay for extended periods of time as his relationship with his father was marked by frequent conflict, especially when Cole failed to meet family expectations. Both Teddy and Cole reported these conflicts can escalate to physical violence between each other. Teddy also stated how he did not like taking Cole to Sam's because Cole's grandfather often undermined Teddy's parenting by reversing his discipline decisions regardless of the offense. Cole also described an estranged relationship with his mother and she was not present for any family session conducted with Cole and his family.

Cole was referred through a local community agency for treatment using a team-based approach for polysubstance abuse. Thus, throughout the case example, "we" represents a variety of family counselors working together in Cole's case. Cole has previously received treatment via inpatient, outpatient, and psychiatric services, all of which failed to curtail his substance abuse. During the first team meeting with Cole, he tested positive for multiple substances including opiates, barbiturates, stimulants, and marijuana. During this discussion, Cole appeared sullen and sat quietly as Teddy disclosed how he sneaks out at night to use drugs. When discussing family resources, Cole brightened up and began discussing how much he loved staying out with his uncle Sam on his land as well as spending time with his grandparents. Teddy confirmed that Cole's behavior was better around family. Treatment goals included reducing and eventually, eliminating Cole's substance use, improving Cole's educational performance, and improving relationships between Cole and his family.

Family Unity over Personal Progress

As compared to mainstream American culture that highly values individual achievement, Appalachian culture has been described as collectivistic and primarily values family well-being (Keefe, 1988). Appalachians' definition of family includes both nuclear and extended (e.g., aunts and uncles) family members with a deep sense of loyalty to their families of origin placing the continuity of this institution above everything else (Keefe & Greene, 2005). To Appalachians, the family unit is the most hospitable environment for all family members. Therefore, treatment goals such as self-actualization (Ellis, 1991) and differentiation (Bowen, 1985) could be interpreted as promoting one member above the rest and met with clients' resistance or therapeutic stagnation.

Adopting a cybernetic/systemic epistemology, we viewed Cole's substance abuse in the context of his family system. During the first session with Cole and his father, we reiterated this focus by stating, "We believe the only way we can help is getting an accurate picture of how Cole is with his entire family." Teddy, showing his relief, responded, "I don't think we can stand him leaving again," referring to Cole's stay at the inpatient facility. Through our continued discussion, we outlined Cole's treatment goals to center on his family. Cole then stated he wanted to be a better family member by being more respectful of others.

Taking a family-focused approach with Cole's case allowed the team to expand their understanding of his problematic behaviors and work in ways respectful of Cole and his family. During individual work with Cole, we ensured information from family sessions remain the focus, by discussing specific strategies he could use when he got angry with his father respecting the family structure and cultural values. Such a stance empowered Cole to relate better with his family.

Appalachian Personalism

Appalachians value personalism (Keefe, 1988; Keefe & Greene, 2005), preferring to "get to know" someone before meaningfully engaging them in business or personal dialogue. This is particularly important for therapeutic treatment as many family counselors expect client cooperation based on their credentials alone. This may not be the case with Appalachian families as they may prefer to know a counselor's personality, values, and experience before trusting them with their family secrets and committing to treatment. When working with Appalachian families, the therapeutic relationship is a key factor to successful treatment.

A strong therapeutic relationship may be facilitated in a variety of ways. First, using interpersonal interview methods rather than specific assessment measures can better facilitate the joining process. Next, when possible, engage the client in their own home giving clients a sense of "home-field advantage." While this can be uncomfortable for family counselors accustomed to office-based treatment, in-home therapy can comfort families during treatment. Furthermore, this allows for a more accurate assessment of clients' family dynamics as they are more likely to engage in their everyday behaviors in their natural environment (Lemon et al., 1993).

Finally, as Appalachians are a proud, self-sustaining people, they'll try to "compensate" family counselors by bringing them vegetables from their garden, offering them portions of food if the session takes place during dinner time, or even small acts such as offering coffee during the session. It can be meaningful for the family when family counselors accept these gestures – if ethically appropriate – providing them with a sense of pride and empowerment in the therapeutic process. As Appalachians want to contribute to the process, and not "put anyone out," flatly rejecting all such gestures can come across as being "too good" for them and be detrimental to the therapeutic relationship (Cole, 1988; Helton, 1995; Keefe & Greene, 2005; Lemon et al., 1993; Russ, 2010).

Initially Teddy and Cole would not meet with the team at Uncle Sam's home with Teddy stating, "I'll have to check on that. Everybody is pretty busy out there" when the idea was brought up. We noticed Teddy would often make and offer us coffee during session, which they would refuse due to agency guidelines. We recognized we were presenting ourselves in a manner based on our professional value set. Following Minuchin's (1974) stance of joining the family system by accommodation, or adopting their language, values, and style, we shifted our approach and began dressing more casually and opening sessions with small talk Teddy and Cole valued. We also accepted Teddy's coffee during these conversations, an act supported by our supervisor, and noticed Cole and Teddy using humor in describing one another and their problems, a tactic we adopted later in treatment. After two sessions, Teddy invited us to Uncle Sam's house to meet the family. Matching the personalism displayed by Cole and his family created the opportunity for connection. Teddy's permission for us to meet his extended family provided us an opportunity to assess the interactional dynamics of the entire family and a more complete picture of Cole's behavior.

Distrust of Outsiders

Appalachians have a natural distrust of outsiders, especially state and/or government workers (Brown & May, 2005; Keefe, 1988; Lohri-Posey, 2006; Owens, Richerson, Murphy, Jageleweksi, & Rossi, 2007), stemming from previous exploitations of Appalachian natives (e.g., coal mining, lumber, textile industries, strip mining, logging and many others; Helton, 1995). Distrust towards family counselors should be viewed as a natural mechanism to protect one's family from exploitation and not as paranoia or lack of engagement. Although it is time consuming, once one earns the trust of an Appalachian family, they can be fiercely loyal and open to a variety of therapeutic interventions (Cole, 1988; Denham, 2016; Keefe 1988; Keefe & Greene, 2005; Lemon et al., 1993; Russ, 2010).

Assessing trust in the therapeutic relationship with an Appalachian client can be difficult as they are often non-confrontational in nature and will go to great lengths not to offend others, including those that they distrust. One of the most visible signs of distrust may be the family's lack of follow through with directives and interventions, reluctance to discuss sensitive topics, and even missing appointments citing issues beyond their control (e.g., sick family members, car problems, or other problems requiring immediate attention). This was the case with Cole and his family during previous treatment attempts prior to our involvement. Previous family counselors cited Cole as unmotivated to change, increasing Cole's family distrust in counseling.

After becoming more personable with Cole and Teddy, we meet with members of Cole's extended family. The first family session included Cole, Teddy, Cole's grandmother, grandfather, and uncle Sam. Following previous success, we engaged in small personable talk while coffee was made and served to everyone. When the discussion turned from small talk to treatment, we validated Cole's family's previous experiences, respectfully making the covert family distrust towards counselors overt. The family stated they were hurt when Cole left for inpatient treatment in another part of the state and thought it wrong for the counselors to "coerce" Teddy into making Cole go. We took the opportunity to apologize to the family stating, "Sometimes we get so concerned about our clients we can't see the forest for the trees. It is never our intent to put Cole and his loved ones through more emotional pain. We are actually hoping it would be possible to meet here at your family's convenience to continue his treatment at home rather than a stuffy office or another facility." The family agreed but stated, "It's hard to get behind this since we haven't seen any improvement in Cole."

Cole's family did not trust us to fully participate in treatment until Cole improved, and at the same time, meaningful progress with Cole was unlikely unless his family participated. Proceeding under these circumstances would have significantly reduced treatment effectiveness (Watzlawick et al., 1967). To escape this double bind, we used a paradoxical intervention from strategic therapy (Haley, 1987) and encouraged Cole's family not to trust us with anything significant until they felt we were trustworthy and able to help them meet their goals. We validated the family's suspicions of treatment and asked they work on something small first to test if they could trust us more. The family agreed with Teddy stating he wanted to work on managing his emotions better in interacting with and over his ex-wife as well as get a part-time job to help cover costs his disability did not cover.

Through working with Teddy, his family began to see some change in how he was responding to certain situations and began to trust us with the family secrets. It was soon revealed that Cole was not Teddy's biological son, rather his real father was Teddy's brother who experienced a "bad acid trip" and was permanently institutionalized. Teddy also revealed that Cole's biological father was a result of an affair Cole's grandmother had and pointed out his grandfather's treatment of Cole reflects guilt from how he treated Cole's biological father growing up. This information, revealing of the family dynamics, might not have been obtained if we did not address Cole's family's natural distrust of us.

Fatalism

Appalachians can often appear fatalistic, expressing feelings of hopelessness about current issues, a resignation of future events, and a lack of optimism for successful outcomes (Denham, 2016). Fatalism is also connected to the religiosity and spirituality of the Appalachian population. Many Appalachians attribute their problems to "fate" or "God's will," finding value in the struggle and accept them with little resistance. Family counselors working with Appalachians displaying these fatalistic beliefs should actively look for ways to engage clients in dialogue highlighting their strengths.

For example, in a family session with a 17-year-old male displaying aggressive behaviors at school, mom stated, "He's just like his father at his age, only God can change that boy," connecting his behavior to his father who was incarcerated at the time of the session. These statements suggest a sense of hopelessness about behavioral change. The family counselor inquired about the characteristics of the boy's father attractive to her when they first met. She described the father as "strong," "confident," and "fearless in taking risks." Using these descriptions, the family counselor discussed how she could show her son how to be appropriately strong and confident, as well as being fearless in taking risks of being restrained during moments of calamity. Working in this manner helped mom see the influence she had on her son even though he displayed traits "just like his father as his age."

Cole and his family frequently took positions reflecting a fatalistic view of Cole's behaviors. Over the course of treatment, Cole relapsed many times, including sneaking out of the apartment complex and returning home inebriated from parties. During a session after one such occasion occurred, Teddy discussed how much Cole was like his biological father and framed Cole's behaviors as unchangeable, stating, "He's going to do what he's going to do. Maybe God has a plan where Cole has to go through this first." At this point, instead of challenging Teddy about how his beliefs as inaccurate or unhelpful, we decided to expand upon them using a systemic reframe from MRI brief therapy, applying the same principles and beliefs Teddy stated for a different, alternate frame representing more empowerment for Teddy (Gehart, 2014; Watzlawick et al., 1974). The therapist stated, "I think you're right, Teddy. I remember hearing a story about how refiners would have to hold freshly mined gold in fire to purify it; getting all the impurities out. They sit and stare because if it's in the fire for too long it would be destroyed. Cole needs you to pull him out when he's getting roasted by these nasty experiences. You're the refiner in this situation, Teddy." Teddy quipped, "Man, that's deep." Together, we shifted his statements from being hopeless and powerless to an empowered parent. By presenting Teddy with an alternative interpretation of his beliefs, we gained an opportunity to discuss Teddy's need to appropriately intervene when Cole began to drift towards relapse.

Conclusion and Recommendations

After many ups and downs, Cole's behaviors, and Teddy's ability to parent him, improved forging a stronger relationship between the two. These goals were only achieved by respecting their Appalachian culture and using culturally sensitive interventions designed to elicit their cooperation. Taken together, the four cultural traits discussed above – family unity over personal progress, Appalachian personalism, distrust of outsiders, and fatalism – helped us to collaborate with Cole's family effectively. We conclude by encouraging the reader to further explore Appalachian culture by reviewing the recommended resources accompanying this chapter to help expand one's therapeutic knowledge in working with Appalachian families.

Note

1 Cole is a pseudonym to protect his confidentiality and the dialogue given throughout the chapter is not verbatim, but rather a composite of our experience with him.

References

Appalachian Regional Commission. (n.d.). Poverty rates, 2010–2014. Retrieved from www.arc.gov/reports/custom_report.asp?REPORT_ID=64.

Bowen, M. (Ed.) (1985). *Family therapy in clinical practice*. Lanham, MD: Rowman & Littlefield Publishers.

Brown, J., & May, B. (2005). Rural older Appalachian women's formal patterns of care. *Southern Online Journal of Nursing Research*, 6(2), 1–21.
Cole, C. (1988). Appalachian family therapy. In S. Keefe (Ed.), *Appalachian mental health* (pp. 175–187). Lexington, KY: University Press of Kentucky.
Denham, S. A. (2016). Does a culture of Appalachia truly exist? *Journal of Transcultural Nursing*, 27(2), 94–102.
Duncan, C. M. (2001). Social capital in America's poor rural communities. In S. Saegert, J. P. Thompson, & M. R. Warren (Eds.), *Social capital and poor communities* (pp. 60–88). New York:Russell Sage.
Ellis, A. (1991). Achieving self-actualization: The rational-emotive approach. *Journal of Social Behavior and Personality*, 6(5), 1–18.
Foster, G. S., & Hummel, R. L. (1997). Wham, bam, thank you, Sam: Critical dimensions of the persistence of hillbilly caricatures. *Sociological Spectrum*, 17(2), 157–176.
Foster, S. W. (1988). *The past is another country: Representation, historical consciousness, and resistance in the Blue Ridge*. Berkeley, CA: University of California Press.
Gehart, D. (2014). *Mastering competencies in family therapy: A practical approach to theory and clinical case documentation* (2nd ed.). Belmont, CA: Brooks/Cole.
Gollnick, D. M., & Chinn, P. C. (1998). *Multicultural education in a pluralistic society* (5th ed.). Columbus, OH: Merrill/Prentice-Hall.
Gore, J. S., Sheppard, A., Waters, M., Jackson, J., & Brubaker, R. (2016). Cultural differences in seeking mental health counseling: The role of symptom severity and type in Appalachian Kentucky. *Journal of Rural Mental Health, 40*(1), 63–76. doi:10.1037/rmh0000041.
Haley, J. (1987). *Problem-solving therapy*. San Francisco, CA: Jossey-Bass.
Hayden, W. (2004). Appalachian diversity: African-American, Hispanic/Latino, and other populations. *Journal of Appalachian Studies*, 10(3), 293–306.
Helton, L. (1995). Intervention with Appalachians: Strategies for a culturally specific practice. *Journal of Cultural Diversity*, 2(1), 20–26.
Hendryx, M. (2008). Mental health professional shortage areas in rural Appalachia. *The Journal of Rural Health*, 24(2), 179–182. doi:10.1111/j.1748–0361.2008.00155.x.
Hendryx, M. (2009). Mortality from heart, respiratory, and kidney disease in coal mining areas of Appalachia. *International Archives of Occupational and Environmental Health, 82*(2), 243–249. doi:10.1007/s00420-008-0328-y.
Hendryx, M., Ahern, M. M., & Nurkiewicz, T. R. (2007). Hospitalization patterns associated with Appalachian coal mining. *Journal of Toxicology and Environmental Health, Part A, 70*(24), 2064–2070. doi:10.1080/15287390701601236.
Hendryx, M., & Zullig, K. J. (2009). Higher coronary heart disease and heart attack morbidity in Appalachian coal mining regions. *Preventive Medicine, 49*(5), 355–359. doi:10.1016/j.ypmed.2009.09.011.
Jackson, H., Judd, F., Komiti, A., Fraser, C., Murray, G., Robins, G., … Wearing, A. (2007). Mental health problems in rural contexts: What are the barriers to seeking help from professional providers? *Australian Psychologist*, 42(2), 147–160.
Keefe, S. (1988). Appalachian Americans: The formulation of "relunctant" ethnics. In G. Campbell (Ed.), *Many Americas: Critical perspectives on race, racism, and ethnicity* (pp. 129–153). Dubuque, IA: Kendall Hunt Publishing.
Keefe, S. (2000, March). Mountain identity and the global society in a rural Appalachian county. Paper presented at the Center for Ethnicity and Gender in Appalachia's National Conference, Huntington, WV.

Keefe, S., & Greene, S. (2005). Mental health therapy for Appalachian clients. In S. Keefe (Ed.), *Appalachian cultural competency: A guide for medical, mental health, and social service professionals* (pp. 299–314). Knoxville, TN: University of Tennessee Press.

Keeney, B. P. (1979). Ecosystemic epistemology: An alternative paradigm for diagnosis. *Family process*, 18(2), 117–129.

Keeney, B. P., & Ross, J. M. (1985). *Mind in therapy: Constructing systemic family therapies.* New York:Basic Books.

Keller, S. M., & Helton, L. R. (2010). Culturally competent approaches for counseling urban Appalachian clients: An exploratory case study. *Journal of Social Service Research, 36* (2), 142–150. doi:10.1080/01488370903578090.

Lemon, S. D., Newfield, N. A., & Dobbins, J. E. (1993). Culturally sensitive family therapy in Appalachia. *Journal of Systemic Therapies, 12*(4), 8–26. doi:10.1521/jsyt.1993.12.4.8.

Liddle, H. A. (1983). Diagnosis and assessment in family therapy: A comparative analysis of six schools of thought. In B. P. Keeney (Ed.), *Diagnosis and assessment in family therapy* (pp. 1–33). Rockville, MD: Aspen.

Lohri-Posey, B. (2006). Middle-aged Appalachians living with Diabetes Mellitus: A family affair. *Family & Community Health*, 29(3), 214–220.

Minuchin, S. (1974). *Families and family therapy*. Cambridge, MA: Harvard University Press.

Owens, J. S., Richerson, L., Murphy, C. E., Jageleweski, A., & Rossi, L. (2007). The parent perspective: Informing the cultural sensitivity of parenting programs in rural communities. *Child and Youth Care Forum*, 36(5), 179–194.

Polaha, J., DaltonIII, W. T., & Allen, S. (2011). The prevalence of emotional and behavior problems in pediatric primary care serving rural children. *Journal of Pediatric Psychology, 36*(6), 652–660. doi:10.1093/jpepsy/jsq116.

Pollard, K., & Jacobsen, L. A. (2011). The Appalachian region in 2010: A census data overview. (Contract No. CO-16506–16509). Retrieved from Appalachian Regional Commission website: www.prb.org/pdf12/appalachia-census-chartbook-2011.pdf.

Pollard, K., & Jacobsen, L. A. (2017). The Appalachian region: A data overview from the 2011–2015 American community survey. (Contract No. CO-18662–18616). Retrieved from Appalachian Regional Commission website: www.arc.gov/assets/research_reports/DataOverviewfrom2011to2015ACS.pdf.

Poole, K., Romitti, M., White, M., Feser, E., Mix, T., Gutschow, S., ... Manzi, P. (2015). Appalachia then and now: Examining changes to the Appalachian region since 1965. Retrieved from Appalachian Regional Commission website: www.arc.gov/research/researchreportdetails.asp?REPORT_ID=113.

Russ, K. A. (2010). Working with clients of Appalachian culture. Retrieved from www.counseling.org/resources/library/VISTAS/2010-V-Online/Article_69.pdf.

Watzlawick, P., Bavelas, J. B., & Jackson, D. D. (1967). *Pragmatics of human communication: A study of interactional patterns, pathologies, and paradoxes*. New York: W. W. Norton & Company.

Watzlawick, P., Weakland, J. H., & Fisch, R. (1974). *Change: Principles of problem formation and problem resolution*. New York: W. W. Norton & Company.

Zhang, Z., Infante, A., Meit, M., English, N., Dunn, M., & Bowers, K. (2008). *An analysis of mental health and substance abuse disparities & access to treatment services in the Appalachian region*. Washington, D.C.: Appalachian Regional Commission.

Recommended Appalachian Resources

Billings, D. B., Norman, G., & Ledford, K. (2001). *Back talk from Appalachia: Confronting stereotypes*. Lexington, KY: University Press of Kentucky.

Edwards, G. T., Asbury, J. A., & Cox, R. L. (Eds.) (2006). *A handbook to Appalachia*. Knoxville, TN: University of Tennessee Press.

Keefe, S. (Ed.) (2005). *Appalachian cultural competency: A guide for medical, mental health, and service professionals*. Knoxville, TN: University of Tennessee Press.

Lemon, S. D., Newfield, N. A., & Dobbins, J. E. (1993). Culturally sensitive family therapy in Appalachia. *Journal of Systemic Therapies, 12*(4), 8–26. doi:10.1521/jsyt.1993.12.4.8.

Russ, K. A. (2010). Working with clients of Appalachian culture. Retrieved from www.counseling.org/resources/library/VISTAS/2010-V-Online/Article_69.pdf.

Family Therapy Recommended Resources

Minuchin, S., & Fishman, H. C. (2009). *Family therapy techniques*. Cambridge, MA: Harvard University Press.

Minuchin, P., Colapinto, J., & Minuchin, S. (2007). *Working with families of the poor* (2nd ed.). New York:Guilford Press.

Watzlawick, P., Weakland, J. H., & Fisch, R. (1974). *Change: Principles of problem formation and problem resolution*. New York: W. W. Norton & Company.

INDEX

For Product Safety Concerns and Information please contact our EU
representative GPSR@taylorandfrancis.com
Taylor & Francis Verlag GmbH, Kaufingerstraße 24, 80331 München, Germany

www.ingramcontent.com/pod-product-compliance
Ingram Content Group UK Ltd.
Pitfield, Milton Keynes, MK11 3LW, UK
UKHW021306260926
475702UK00048B/741
9780815379980